How to Prevent Your Next Heart Attack

How to Prevent Your Next Heart Attack

John K. Vyden, M.D., F.A.C.C.

Foreword by H. J. C. Swan, M.D., Ph.D., F.A.C.C., M.A.C.P.
Past President of the American College of Cardiologists

Prentice Hall Press

To my wife,
Barbara Alexandra Vyden

The ideas, procedures, and suggestions contained in this book are not intended to replace the services of a trained health professional. All matters regarding your health require medical supervision. You should consult your physician before adopting the procedures in this book.

The cases and examples cited in this book are based on actual situations and real people. Names and identifying details have been changed to protect privacy.

Published by Prentice Hall Press
A Division of Simon & Schuster, Inc.
Gulf + Western Building
One Gulf + Western Plaza
New York, NY 10023

PRENTICE HALL PRESS is a registered trademark of Simon & Schuster, Inc.

Library of Congress Cataloging-in-Publication Data

Vyden, John K., 1933–
How to prevent your next heart attack.

1. Heart—Infarction—Patients—Rehabilitation.
2. Heart—Infarction—Prevention. I. Title.
RC685.I6V93 1988 616.1′24 87-17506
ISBN 0-13-430661-9

Designed by Barbara Bert

Manufactured in the United States of America

10 9 8 7 6 5 4 3 2 1

First Edition

Acknowledgments

My wife, Barbara Alexandra Vyden, has been magnificently involved in the writing of this book from inception to publication. When I faltered, she was there, encouraging, helping, and being optimistic. Without her great love and support, this opus would never have reached its conclusion. Our children, Sarah, David, and Christopher, also contributed in their own inimitable and often highly amusing ways.

The Honorable R. Clyde Packer, a close friend from my teenage days in Australia and similarly transplanted to California, suggested that I write this book. Thank you, Clyde!

I give special acknowledgment to the many superb doctors and nurses who educated me in cardiology and helped me educate others. Among the many, and in a rough chronological order, are: John B. Hickie, A.O., M.B., F.A.C.C.; Ossie B. Tofler, M.B., F.R.A.C.P.; Tom B. Cullity, M.B., F.R.C.P., F.R.A.C.P.; Eliot Corday, M.D., F.A.C.C.; H. J. C. Swan, M.D., Ph.D., F.A.C.C., M.A.C.P.; Harold B. Rose, Sc.D; Robert M. Kass, M.D., F.A.C.C.; Bonnie J. Zimmerman, M.D.; Elaine M. Mickle, R.N.; Susan A. Orzeck, R.N.; and Barbara B. Lunsford, R.N.

My literary agents, Elise Goodman and Jill L. N. Hickson, are two brilliant and extraordinary women. They could not have been more supportive, interested, and helpful to me. My editor at Prentice Hall Press, P. J. Dempsey, provided patience, great insight, and a delightful sense of humor—all when they were needed most. Susan Solomon helped me in critical editing and rewriting of the manuscript. Susan is a gifted wordsmith and a joy to work with. Finally, my thanks go to Kathleen Moloney, the focused gentlewoman who gave of her time and herself in the writing of the final draft of this work.

Contents

Foreword by H. J. C. Swan, M.D. xiii
Introduction xvii

1 Life After a Heart Attack 1

Your Life Expectancy 2
Questions You Should Ask 3
Your Emotions 3
Your Family 5
Choosing a Doctor 7
Second Opinions 12
Support Systems 13

2 Anatomy of a Heart Attack 14

How the Heart Works 14
What Happens During a Heart Attack? 16
What Causes a Heart Attack? 17
How Do You Know if You Have Had a Heart Attack? 19
Early Treatment 21
The Healing Process 22

3 Conditions Related to Heart Attacks 24
Angina 24
Pulmonary Embolism 26
Arrhythmias 27
Congestive Heart Failure 28
Pericarditis 30
Silent Ischemia 30
Mitral Valve Prolapse 31

4 Your Hospital Stay 32
The Cardiac Care Unit 32
Typical CCU Procedures 34
The Step-down Unit 36
Visitors 38
Getting You up and Moving 40
Cardiac Function Tests 41
Hurry up and Wait 46
Overtesting 47

5 Surgery and Other Cardiac Procedures 48
Angioplasty 49
Thrombolysis 50
Bypass Surgery 50
Pacemakers 53
Heart Transplants 55
Artificial Hearts and Trans-Species Transplants 56
Lasers and Beyond 57

6 The Heart Patient's Pharmacy 59
Beta Blockers 60
Cardiotonic Glycosides 61
Antiarrhythmics 62
Nitrates 62
Diuretics 65
Anticoagulants 66
Calcium Channel Blockers 67

Other Medications 68
Four Important Pieces of Advice 68
The Future of Medication 69
Chart of Heart Medications 69

7 Outpatient Cardiac Rehabilitation Programs 75

What They Do 76
How to Choose a Program 77
When, How Long, and How Much? 79
Personnel 79
Some Good News 79

8 Leaving the Hospital 81

9 The Convalescent Phase 84

What Is Happening Physically 85
Game Plan for Convalescence 86
Ground Rules for Convalescence 88
Body Mechanics 90
Energy Conservation 91
Household Activities 92
Social Activities 93
Exercise 94

10 Risk Factors 98

Uncontrollables 99
Controllables 100

11 Sex and Your Heart 116

Myths About Sex 118
Resuming Sexual Activity 119

12 Food and Your Heart 122
Basic Nutrition 123
Calories 123
Protein 124
Carbohydrates 124
Fats 125
Cholesterol and Triglycerides 127
Water 129
Salt 129
Other Minerals 130
Vitamins 131

13 How to Lose Weight 141
Why We Gain Weight 141
Fad Diets 142
The Best Diet Program 143
Setting Goals 144
Shopping, Meal Planning, and Cooking 144
Social Occasions 146
When You Slip 147
Support Systems 147
Exercise 148
How I Kicked the Ice-cream Habit 149

14 The Conditioning Phase 152
Introducing METs 154
Taking Your Pulse 157
Your Target Heart Rate 157
How to Exercise 160
How Often to Exercise 161
Beating the Heat 162
Choosing the Right Exercise 162
Traveling 171
Saying "No" 171
Returning to Work 172

15 The Psychology of Healing 175

Conquering Depression 176
Denial 178
Projection 180
Obsessive Compulsion 181
The Nagging Problem 181
Medication 183
Professional Assistance 183

16 Money Matters 186

Financing Cardiac Rehabilitation 187
Family Finances 188
Workers' Compensation 188
Disability and Retirement 189

17 Planning for an Emergency 191

Planning Ahead 192
Heart Attack Warning Signs 193
Dangers of Denial 194

18 Maintenance 195

Exercise 196
Your New Target Heart Rate 197
Weight 199
Continuing Education 199
Illness 200
Support Systems 201

19 Rehabilitating the Spirit 202

Cardiac Glossary 204
Recommended Reading 211
Index 214

Foreword

In contrast to the victims of many other diseases, the heart attack victim has available a number of positive options for achieving a normal or near-normal life span and, perhaps more important, a quality of life that remains satisfying. For the survivor of a heart attack, two fundamental medical issues are critical—the amount of actual damage to the heart muscle and the underlying obstructions due to disease in the larger coronary arteries. The magnitude of heart muscle destruction (or perhaps, more correctly, the amount of healthy heart muscle remaining), determines the capability of the heart as a pump to continue to perform its essential bodily function. The presence, location, and severity of the narrowing of the arteries, other than the vessel that recently closed off, are principal determinants of the occurrence of further heart attacks and also of chest pains, shortness of breath, or other troublesome symptoms, or as we now know, disturbances of heart function without chest discomfort (termed *silent ischemia*).

The first prerequisite for recovery is the intelligent, informed participation of both the heart attack victim and the partner, spouse, or person closest to the victim. The initial reaction of both parties is usually fear, followed by anxiety resulting in differing degrees of depression, or not infrequently, a relinquishing of responsibility to a third party for all aspects of the victim's future health. Others tend to ignore the issue completely and take their chances. Many patients and families just don't want any reminder of the fact that the victim has indeed had a heart attack.

Dr. Vyden's book is directed to the heart attack victim and spouse as an integral part of the "team" approach to the comprehensive management of coronary heart disease. His target is clearly defined: the survivor and spouse. The information is sufficiently detailed to allow the reader to appreciate the benefits that can be offered to the heart attack victim at this time in history. He makes it clear that the available resources of physicians, nurses, rehabilitation experts, and the like is impressive, but they are all useless unless the heart attack victim participates fully and completely in his or her own recovery. Intelligent participation also means questioning the physician, dietitian, physical therapist, and psychiatrist. I regard this process as similar to inquiry of an accountant or bank manager. While it may be unpleasant to recognize that an overdraft is imminent, prior knowledge allows one to make appropriate responses and adjustments.

Dr. Vyden's approach is fundamentally practical, based on extensive experience in the field of cardiac rehabilitation. Wisely, he points out that there is much more to the optimal care of the heart attack victim than risk-factor reductions, diet, and exercise. In particular, he underscores the need for attending to warning signs that may suggest a high probability of further troubles as well as the need for adequate and truly meaningful communication with the responsible medical staff. Your doctor is the captain of the team, he says, but be sure that he or she is indeed in charge. The patient's attitude is frequently based on his confidence in the competence of his chosen physician. If your confidence in your doctor is low, then switch doctors. If the physician is an alarmist, seek a more balanced view.

At this time in the development of the science of diagnostic investigation and invasive treatment, every patient should be considered for evaluation after a first or second heart attack. In some, angiography and invasive therapy may indeed not be justified by the underlying clinical situation; in others, it may be mandatory. Dr. Vyden's approach as outlined in this volume is a balanced one. It reflects the immense potential for heart attack victims to participate meaningfully in those decisions that affect survival and the quality of life in the years to come.

As a psalmist put it, "I am fearfully and wonderfully made." But from time to time, restorative measures further these human characteristics. The first step, that of intelligent, informed participation, must be taken by the heart attack victim and spouse. *How to Prevent Your Next Heart Attack* shows them the way.

—H. J. C. Swan, M.D., Ph.D., F.A.C.C., M.A.C.P.

Introduction

Some of the most upbeat, cheerful individuals I know are those in a cardiac rehabilitation program. That may sound peculiar, but if you think about it for a moment, you'll understand why. These are people who have suffered one of life's most frightening experiences—a heart attack—and lived to tell about it. They're truly happy to be alive.

If you are just beginning to recover from your heart attack, chances are you're not feeling all that great. You may find it hard to believe that others who have had your disease are now leading normal, even vigorous lives. Believe it. People who work hard at their rehabilitation after a heart attack are nearly always healthier than they were before the incident took place.

What's the secret? Taking an active part in your recovery process. In the past, those recovering from heart attacks assumed a passive role. They lay in bed and let the doctor take care of them, accepting whatever treatment was offered. It isn't like that any more. Today, successful heart patients (note the use of the word *successful*) regard themselves as members of a recovery team. They work with their physicians, nurses, pharmacists, cardiac rehabilitation therapists, and everyone else who is trying to make them well.

The first step in becoming a member of this team is to educate yourself. Learn what you can do to make yourself better and to prolong your life. Now I don't mean that you should enroll in medical school, but I do think that you should learn a little something about anatomy and physiology, at least as it applies to the recovering heart patient.

And that's what this book is all about. Think of *How to Prevent Your Next Heart Attack* as your own cardiac rehabilitation guide. It will show you the way, from your first day in the hospital, through the cardiac care unit, through the myriad tests and possibly surgery, through convalescence and the conditioning phase, right up to maintenance. Along the way I've tried to cover every detail of cardiac care and treatment, including medication, related health conditions that may develop, and doctor-patient relations.

Since one of the most important aspects of cardiac rehabilitation is emotional recovery, I address that as well. Just as you'll probably have to make a few changes in the physical dimension of your life—exercising your muscles, for instance—you may well have to think about giving your emotions a bit of a workout too. I've included some advice on reducing and handling stress—a malady of the modern age that often contributes to heart problems—and I talk about fear, confusion, anger, and guilt, emotions that are common to almost every patient and family.

As the most active members of your support network, your family will play a critical part in your recovery. They, too, should be encouraged to learn more about the causes and treatment of heart disease. Give them this book to read. Even if they don't want to read it from cover to cover, persuade them to read the sections on nagging, worrying, finances, and sex. Discuss this book with your doctors, too. They will be glad to know that you're taking an active interest in your condition, and they may be willing to emphasize certain points that apply specifically to you. Then, if it's not too dog-eared, let your friends see this book. Again, they won't necessarily want to commit the entire thing to memory, but they will welcome the opportunity to know what you're going through. (Besides, if they had any idea what that cigarette or that triple chocolate sundae was doing to your heart, they'd stop encouraging you to indulge.)

Please understand that *How to Prevent Your Next Heart Attack* is not meant to take the place of a personal relationship between you and your doctor or you and the staff of your cardiac rehabilitation center. Nothing can do that. This book is meant to reinforce what you learn from them, and perhaps to refresh your memory.

I won't say that the time ahead of you will be easy. There will be frustrations, setbacks, and emotional lows along the way. But I will say that you're on the right track. With determination and effort you're going to get healthy and live a long, happy life. Remember, you're one of the lucky ones.

To the readers of this book, the very best of health.

1

Life After a Heart Attack

Congratulations! You are now a certified survivor. You have had one of life's most terrifying experiences—a heart attack—and you lived through it. You proved that in the natural selection process of life, the survival of the fittest, you had what it takes. Now the question to ask yourself is: Do I have what it takes to stay alive?

Of course, you have many other questions as well: Do I have the right doctor? What is a heart attack, anyway? When can I have sex? Do I have to quit smoking? Is it all the fried eggs I've been eating that put me here? Will I ever work or play golf again? Am I going to die?

And those are just the beginning. Don't be embarrassed about having so many questions. This is your time not only for rejoicing in your good fortune but also for learning all you can about staying healthy from now on. And that means getting rid of unnecessary fears and misconceptions about what happened to you and what your future is likely to hold.

So let's get started.

YOUR LIFE EXPECTANCY

The question that I (and every other doctor I know) am most frequently asked by a heart attack patient is, "How long am I going to live?" Unfortunately it's probably also the hardest to answer. In fact, there is no definite answer to this question. Doctors are not God (though occasionally both patients and doctors may like to think they are). Doctors can help extend your life; they cannot determine precisely how long it will be.

However, there are certain hints that give us some insight. First, if you are having a heart attack and think you are dying, you are probably not. The majority of deaths from heart attacks occurs in the first 15 minutes, so if you've had a lot of time to worry, the critical period is over, and you will most likely be okay. A general rule: If you are alive after 15 minutes, the odds of staying alive are markedly in your favor. Moreover, if you're still alive after 48 hours, the chances are excellent that you will soon be going home from the hospital.

The logical follow-up question is, "But now that I've had my heart attack and gone home, is it possible to know—perhaps in terms of years—how long I can expect to go on living?" It is safe to say that many heart attack patients can expect to live at least another 20 years. That is, if you are fifty years old now, you will probably live well into your seventies. Many of you will live to be even older, and you won't necessarily die of heart disease.

As we approach the 1990s, the rate of death from heart attack is beginning to fall slightly, from 38 percent of the population to 36 percent, but even a slight drop is encouraging. We can't be sure what accounts for the decrease in fatalities. Perhaps it's because people have been alerted to the dangers of smoking and obesity, or maybe it's due to the advances in drugs, surgery, and cardiac rehabilitation. But the rate *is* declining.

Medical science is moving forward so rapidly in the areas of diagnosis, management, and treatment of heart disease (through both surgery and medication) that it is impossible to say with certainty how survival rates will be affected over the long run. We can say, however, that the outlook is brightening each year. These new procedures and medications, unheard of even a couple of years ago, have already been very beneficial to heart patients.

Even as you read these words, progress is being made. All around the world, the best and brightest minds are working in hospitals and universities, looking for cures for heart disease. Some of their work may well be completed in time to help you.

QUESTIONS YOU SHOULD ASK

While we're on the subject of the most commonly asked questions, here is a list of the ones you should ask right away if you've had a heart attack—in the emergency room or as soon after that as possible.

1. What happened to me?
2. What caused my heart attack?
3. How many of my coronary arteries are affected?
4. Do I have any complications?
5. Can I expect a return of the complications?
6. Do I need a stress test?
7. Do I need cardiac catheterization?
8. Do I need medication? If so, what kind? What will the side effects be?
9. Do I need surgery?
10. Is it going to happen again?
11. What should I do if it does?

YOUR EMOTIONS

If you've just had a heart attack, you have probably been asked, "How are you feeling?" by doctors, nurses, family, and friends, more times than you care to count. Most likely, you have answered your well-wishers with a few short words and then moved on to another subject. If you do give a longer answer, it's almost always about your physical condition: You're drowsy, restless, warm, thirsty. If you're like a great many heart attack patients, you wouldn't dream of telling your visitors about your state of mind.

Chances are it has always been easier for you to talk about your physical condition than your emotional state. This is quite common. As children, many of us were taught to keep our feelings private. As a result, we keep our emotions bottled up inside, trying to ignore them instead of handling them intelligently. Researchers have discovered that your emotional status can influence your susceptibility to heart attack and the speed and outcome of your recovery once a heart attack has occurred. For obvious reasons, now is an excellent time to reverse some of those childhood habits. It's time to deal sensibly with your emotions.

How do you handle your emotions more intelligently? A good way to begin is by asking yourself these four important questions:

1. Am I prepared to confront some very personal issues in my life?
2. Am I prepared to probe my true feelings about myself, my family, and my career?
3. Will I be able to admit that I'll have to make some changes?
4. Will I have the tenacity to follow through with these changes for the rest of my life?

Naturally, you may be uncomfortable with the idea of working on your emotional recovery, especially if you have been the "strong, silent type" for most of your life. Do not shy away from the challenge, though. Remember that anything worthwhile takes time, and surely there's nothing more worthwhile than prolonging your life.

If you are reading this section soon after your heart attack, you are probably feeling less in control of your emotions than usual. This condition is called *emotional flooding*. A veritable wave of emotions is threatening to engulf you: fear, anxiety, sadness, guilt, anger, and a whole host of other mental woes. You're afraid of dying or losing your job or even missing a payment on the house; you're feeling guilty about smoking and overeating; you're anxious about leaving your wife alone at home or missing your son's graduation.

It may be small comfort, but understand that these feelings are normal, and they are also controllable. (See chapter 15 for details on the psychology of healing.) If you are willing to make the effort, you can stop your emotional flood without drowning. If you're like most of my patients, you'll end up feeling more positive about yourself than you have in years.

YOUR FAMILY

It is often said that the heart attack experience upsets a patient's family more than it upsets the patient. Why? They've had a terrible scare. Although you may be feeling fine, your brush with death may have deeply frightened your spouse, children, parents, siblings, close friends, lovers. For instance, your children may be terrified of losing a provider of love, security, and guidance. Your spouse may fear losing a loving partner and at the same time dread the prospect of becoming the family's sole provider (both emotionally and financially). Your friends may suddenly realize that the bond of friendship will not go on forever.

Although you are likely to be understandably preoccupied with your own feelings, try to remember that the doubts and fears of the people who love you are just as serious and just as important as your own. As you work toward improving your emotional and physical condition after a heart attack, keep in mind that those close to you must also have time to recover.

Often you can all work together. The first step in the process is education; if you make the effort to become more knowledgeable about heart disease, you can work to separate myths from reality, fears from truths. Reading this book together is a good start. Group counseling may help everyone recognize and cope with the fears and other emotions that may hamper the recovery process.

Sometimes togetherness doesn't work. Those close to you are individuals, with their own unique coping mechanisms and personalities. Each may react to a crisis in a completely different manner and require some individual type of counseling. For example, a spouse or child may become severely depressed, even though you have resolved to maintain a positive attitude. Or someone close to you may become overly protective during your recovery even as you strive for independence. Whatever the situation, understanding one another's reactions and needs and keeping the lines of communication open are essential. This is not the time for family squabbles.

I'm certainly not recommending a coronary as part of marriage counseling, but I have seen many families brought closer together by a heart attack. One of my patients was an alcoholic who suffered from angina. Mostly because of his drinking, his marriage had been rocky for years. His wife had tried to work things out, but she was just about at the end of her rope.

Then her husband had a serious heart attack. When he was in the hospital, he had to stop drinking. By the time he was ready to go home, with the support and encouragement of his wife, he vowed never to take a drink again. The day he left the hospital he went to his first Alcoholics Anonymous meeting. Five years later, he still goes to meetings, and their marriage is going strong.

CHOOSING A DOCTOR

Aside from yourself and your loved ones, no one influences your recovery more than your doctor. Consequently, it is imperative that right from the start, you feel confident about the kind of advice and care your physician can provide.

How do you know if your physician is right for you? Unfortunately, there is no tried-and-true formula for choosing a doctor, just as there is no formula for picking a husband or wife. However, there are some important points to think about.

The most important consideration is the level of care you will be needing. (The physicians and staff who are supervising your case during the first few days after your heart attack should be able to tell you this.) Many heart attack patients can be quite comfortably cared for by a general practitioner who is knowledgeable about heart disease, but others will be better off seeing a physician with a higher level of specialization. Most likely this would be an internist who specializes in (or concentrates on) treating heart attack patients.

A qualified internist is someone who has passed the examination of the American Board of Internal Medicine. (You will find this qualification imprinted either on the physician's letterhead or on the diploma hanging in the office.) Most board-certified internists also have the initials F.A.C.P. after their names, which means that they have joined and become Fellows of the American College of Physicians.

If a still higher area of specialization is desirable, you may want to be treated by a cardiologist, who is a physician specifically trained in heart care. These physicians have completed additional years of specialized education in cardiology and passed the Board of Cardiovascular Disease. Most board-certified cardiovascular specialists join and become Fellows of the American College of Cardiology and are identified by the initials F.A.C.C. after their names. Still others are fellows working with the American Heart Association. By the way, don't be overly dazzled by the initials after a doctor's name. Most doctors are entitled to use many more than they actually put on their business cards or office walls.

Since there are only about 12,000 cardiologists in the United States, naturally not every hospital has a cardiologist on staff; you'll usually be able to find one in a city with a population of 50,000 or more. Even if it involves a certain amount of trouble and expense, I think, everyone who has had a heart attack should be thoroughly examined by a cardiologist at least once. Any follow-up treatment can be monitored by a general practitioner or internist.

As you make your decision about which doctor to use, one of the concerns you may have is which hospital the doctor uses. There are many types of hospitals in the United States, ranging from quite small (fewer than 100 beds) to quite large (more than 600 beds). Some are for-profit facilities headed by large health care organizations (usually called *proprietary* or *investor-owned* institutions). Others operate on a nonprofit basis, meaning that funds raised are redirected back to the facility for improvement of its services. Still others have religious affiliations, although patient care is usually nondenominational.

University teaching hospitals are those large institutions affiliated with a major university. Here, undergraduate and postgraduate medical students receive their training and learn about the latest advancements in their field. The medical profession usually looks upon these hospitals as the most technically advanced, since the staff will probably include several regional or national authorities working at the forefront of medical research.

The Doctor–Patient Relationship

Once you have decided on the type of doctor you need, it's time to begin cultivating a good relationship with him or her, and that involves establishing complete confidence and trust. Remember, you will be seeing this doctor for a long time on a regular basis during your recovery, and later on you'll be visiting for checkups. Your physician need not be your best friend, but you should at least feel you can talk together openly and comfortably.

Communication between you and your physician is extremely important. Your doctor should not be too rushed to speak with you during—or even between—visits. If you get the feeling you're being hurried out of the office, take a deep breath and say something about it. If you need time to ask questions, say so. And when you're asked questions, don't just answer automatically. For instance, do you immediately shake your head "no" when the physician asks if you are experiencing any pain? If you do, it could be a reaction to your doctor's domineering attitude. This kind of behavior will not help you with your treatment.

Make sure your doctor takes time to explain in simple terms what is happening to you. Under these circumstances, ignorance is definitely not bliss, as can be illustrated by the experience of one of my own patients.

The patient, a middle-aged man, was admitted to the cardiac care unit via the emergency entrance. While in the emergency room, he was told he was having a heart attack and would soon be transferred to the intensive care unit.

Some time later, as the patient's own physician, I came on the scene. When I went to the cardiac care unit to see my patient, I found him severely depressed. When I asked him what was wrong—his heart attack had been mild, and there was no reason for him to be disturbed to this degree—he said he was confused. First they told him in the emergency room that he was having a heart attack. Then, in the cardiac care unit, he was told that he had had a myocardial infarction. "A heart attack is bad enough," he said miserably. "Now I've got to deal with a myocardial infarction!"

I calmed him down by telling him that *myocardial infarction* is the medical term for heart attack.

Granted, you may already know what a myocardial infarction is, but plenty of other terms that your physician may use will undoubtedly sound completely foreign. When that happens, ask for an explanation, especially if it is early in your recovery. The longer you put off asking questions, the more confused and anxious you will become.

Often doctors, nurses, technicians, therapists, and other health professionals will use medical terminology not because they want to make you nervous but because it's the way they're used to speaking to their colleagues. Let them know that they must make the extra effort of providing you with translations, that you are interested in your treatment, and that you expect to be kept informed.

Never be afraid to question why a procedure, test, or medication is being prescribed. Ask for explanations and don't stop asking until you get an answer you understand. If you forget to ask a question during one visit, write it down so you remember next time.

Consider that you may have to interpret what your doctor says to family members or concerned friends. You need to be a virtual information center about your condition. You may even consider bringing someone with you during consultations with your doctor. Many communications problems can be avoided this way.

Think of yourself and your doctor as members of a team. Unless each of you knows what the other is doing, you can't work toward a common goal; in fact, you may be working at cross purposes.

Changing Doctors

No one can be sure of choosing the right physician until seeing and talking with the physician a few times. After the first few sessions with a new doctor, ask yourself the following questions:

1. Does this doctor display technical skill and scientific knowledge?
2. Do I trust this person?
3. Is this doctor a good listener?
4. Does this doctor appreciate me as an individual? Is he or she genuinely interested in my problems?
5. Does this doctor keep good records? Will I be cared for adequately during an absence?
6. Is guidance provided for the nurses, therapists, and other medical professionals involved in my care?

In an ideal world you will answer "yes" to every one of these questions, but it's far more likely that you'll come up with a few "undecideds" or maybe even a "no" or two. Do whatever you can to resolve any conflicts you have with your doctor. If you can't resolve them, give serious thought to finding a new doctor. Be sure you're not changing doctors for the wrong reason, though. Many people blame their doctors for their ill health. I once overheard a patient say to his wife, "If my doctor were any good, I wouldn't have had the heart attack in the first place!" While his reaction is understandable, it's not rational. Don't act in haste.

Don't feel guilty about changing doctors; you aren't the first, and you certainly won't be the last, to do so. When I conducted an informal test among my cardiac rehabilitation patients, I discovered that about 10 percent of all the patients changed doctors in a six-month period.

How do you find another physician? A good first move is to survey the opinions of other physicians in the area. Take the time to make phone calls. Ask these doctors to name the colleagues they would use if they had a heart attack. If you make enough calls, the names of one or two individuals should be repeated.

You may also want to use one of the doctor-referral services available through your County Medical Association, the American Heart Association, or your local hospital. These services will give you a list of several doctors who specialize in heart care. Then ask a friend or family member to help you do some legwork, researching several physicians' credentials through the local library or the AMA. Find out which doctors are active in postgraduate education at a university.

It can't hurt to ask your friends and relatives for their opinions, too. They can usually offer some interesting insights into things that don't show up in a physician's official credentials: "bedside manner," billing procedures, office staff. All of these things will influence how comfortable and confident you will be.

SECOND OPINIONS

Sometimes the impulse to change doctors can be deflected by getting a second opinion. Feel free to do this at any time.

Requesting a second opinion—or even a third if you're especially worried about something—is perfectly legitimate, and it should not be interpreted by your doctor as a vote of no confidence. However, be sure that you're not just looking for a doctor who will give you the opinion you want to hear instead of the one that is best for you. Remember, you and your doctor are partners. There will be some give and take along the way, but it's essential that you feel that you are both working together.

SUPPORT SYSTEMS

Over the next few months, as you begin to recover from the physical trauma you've endured and as you help yourself get better, you're going to need a great deal of support, both physical and psychological. As far as I'm concerned, you should take support anywhere you can get it, from family, friends, co-workers, and health care professionals, such as doctors, nurses, psychiatrists, psychologists, social workers, and psychotherapists. Sometimes the greatest support of all comes from strangers—other heart patients and their families. If you think that meeting other people who have shared an experience similar to yours will be helpful (and I highly recommend it), ask your doctor to make some introductions or recommend an existing support group. As you face life after a heart attack, every bit of support helps.

2
Anatomy of a Heart Attack

Walk into any emergency room and take a look around. You'll probably see a woman about to give birth. You may hear a few crying infants. You may even see an open wound or two. What you may also see on any given day or night is a middle-aged individual who is pale, perhaps ashen, and bathed in sweat. The person is restless and short of breath, and keeps grabbing his chest. When asked about the pain, this patient describes it as incredible pressure, as if his chest is being held in a vise; different from anything ever felt before. The person is probably having a heart attack.

HOW THE HEART WORKS

Your heart is a truly amazing muscle. Only slightly larger than your clenched fist, it keeps a steady beat every moment of your life, continuously supplying blood to all parts of your body. In a single day it will beat approximately 100,000 times and move about 5,000 gallons of blood through the 60,000 miles of blood vessels that form the circulatory system. Most human hearts beat at least 2 billion times, for about 70 years, before anything goes wrong.

One reason for your heart's ability to do so much is its incredibly efficient (but complicated) support system of arteries and veins. The arteries carry the freshly pumped blood containing oxygen and other nutrients away from the heart, and the veins bring back to the heart "used" blood that contains mostly carbon dioxide and waste products. At this point, the blood will again flow through the heart, where it is replenished with life-giving oxygen.

A network of smaller blood vessels supports the arteries and veins. The arteries are supported by smaller branches of blood-carrying vessels called *arterioles.* From each arteriole, a network of fine tubing called *capillaries* reaches out to the surrounding tissue cells. These tissues have extremely thin walls, allowing oxygen and other nutrients in the blood they carry to be absorbed by body tissue—even tissue as far from your heart as your big toe. Capillaries also pick up carbon dioxide and other waste products from these faraway places, carrying them back to vessels called the *venules* and then to the veins that lead to the heart.

I realize that even this simple explanation of the circulatory system may seem complicated, but bear with me, please. If you are to understand what happened to you during your heart attack, you need to know how the heart and its supporting organs function. Let's finish up the story by going back to that big toe.

Having arrived rich with oxygen via an arteriole, the blood brought to the toe then travels through the capillary network, giving off oxygen and collecting carbon dioxide and other waste products. These tiny capillaries then join the venules, which in turn become larger veins. Then the blood goes from a large vein in your foot and up your leg, where it joins other veins from your abdomen and your other leg. At this junction a very important vein, called the *inferior vena cava,* is formed.

The inferior vena cava and a second vein, the *superior vena cava,* are the two veins that lead to the heart. Just as blood containing impurities from the lower body region travels to the heart via the inferior vena cava, blood containing impurities from the upper body region is transported to the heart via the superior vena cava. All this impure blood flows into the heart chamber called the *right atrium,* and the right atrium pumps the blood into the heart's right ventricle. From there the blood is pumped out of the heart, via the pulmonary artery, into the lungs.

Once the blood is in the lungs, the blood's red cells expel carbon dioxide and receive the fresh oxygen inhaled when you breathe. When this exchange is complete, the blood goes back into the heart via the pulmonary vein. First it goes to the heart chamber called the *left atrium* and then to the left ventricle. The left ventricle, which is the biggest of the heart's four pumping chambers, then pumps the fresh blood into the aorta and the major arteries of the body.

From these major arteries the blood travels through a vast arterial network passing through your abdomen, thigh, and leg, to deliver oxygen and nutrients to the big toe once again. Then the whole cycle is repeated.

Blood flows in only one direction—from the lungs, out of the heart, into the largest arteries, and then to the smaller ones. From there it goes into the capillaries, to the tiny veins, and then to larger ones, eventually traveling back into the heart and lungs. Four valves in the heart are responsible for keeping this flow uniform. When these valves are not working, the blood will begin to flow backward, and congestive heart failure may occur.

WHAT HAPPENS DURING A HEART ATTACK?

When the heart stops beating, the whole circulatory system breaks down, and the body tissue is prevented from receiving nutrients. Without these nutrients, the tissues start to die. If the heart stops beating during an attack, it is critical to get it started again as fast as possible, so that those parts of the body particularly sensitive to a lack of oxygen will not be affected. Certain parts of the brain, for instance, will undergo irreversible change and die if deprived of oxygen for just four minutes.

Like the tissue it services, the heart needs its own supply of freshly oxygenated blood to function. The three arteries supplying your heart with this freshly oxygenated blood are called *coronary arteries*. These arteries originate at the junction of the left ventricle and the aorta and divide into smaller branches in order to supply every portion of the heart muscle with blood and oxygen.

If just one coronary artery suddenly becomes blocked, the heart muscle will have difficulty beating, since it is being deprived of some of the oxygen it needs to function. In severe heart attacks, the heart muscle becomes so starved of oxygen, it stops beating altogether. Fortunately there are three major coronary arteries, so if one becomes totally blocked, it is not necessarily fatal.

Blockage of blood flow in one of the coronary arteries is called *myocardial infarction,* the medical term for heart attack. Technically, myocardial infarction refers to the death of a portion of heart muscle due to lack of blood supply.

WHAT CAUSES A HEART ATTACK?

Ironically, while a heart attack is sudden, it is often the result of something that has been going on for decades inside the body—a progressive disease called *atherosclerosis of the coronary arteries*. Atherosclerosis is caused by fatty deposits that build up inside the artery, eventually narrowing the vessel to the point of total obstruction. Think about rust building up inside pipes. A heart attack is caused when the "rust" (fat) deposit becomes so substantial that all blood flow in your body's "pipes" (coronary arteries) suddenly stops.

Keeping this rusty pipe analogy in mind, look at the illustration. This drawing shows coronary arteries that have been narrowed by a slow buildup of fat deposits along their inner lining. This buildup blocks the blood's path, making it difficult for a steady stream of blood to run through. When the arteries are partially blocked (see the circular detail on the right), chest pain, called *angina,* usually occurs. When the buildup completely blocks blood flow or when a blood clot forms in an already narrowed coronary artery (see the circular blowup on the left), the result is a heart attack.

Sometimes a heart attack is caused by *coronary artery spasm.* When it does happen, the spasm stops blood flow in the artery in much the same way the arteries are blocked as a result of atherosclerosis.

Some patients believe that something they just did—arguing or having sexual intercourse or playing tennis—caused

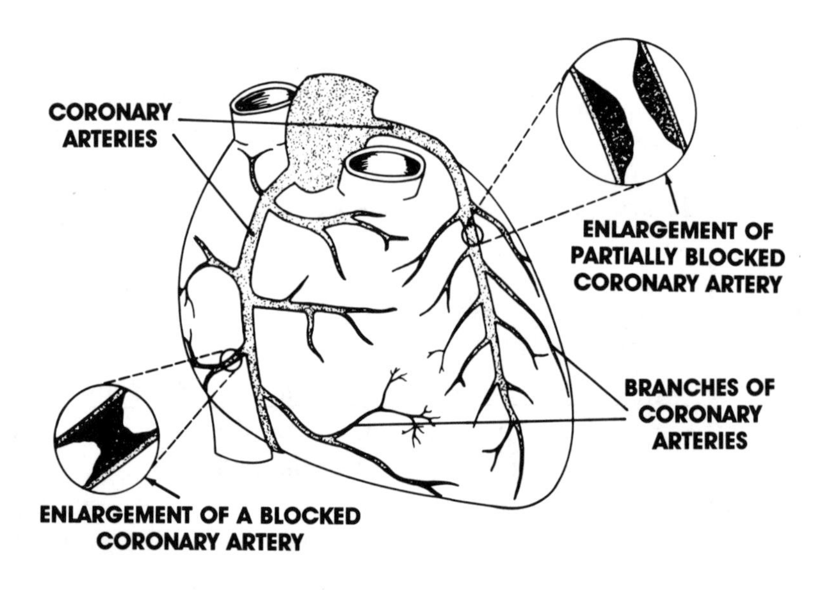

their heart attacks, but this is very rarely true. Atherosclerosis builds up for years and years. You and your family must understand that blaming your heart attack on a sudden, recent action is a misconception that will only cause unnecessary guilt. Remind yourself and explain to others that the argument you had the week of your heart attack had nothing to do with its underlying cause. It will give everyone more peace of mind.

HOW DO YOU KNOW IF YOU HAVE HAD A HEART ATTACK?

The most common symptom associated with heart attack is a squeezing, heaviness, tightness, or crushing pain in the front of the chest. Some patients say it feels as if someone very heavy is sitting on their chest. Discomfort may also be felt in the arms, shoulders, neck, jaw, back, or abdomen. This discomfort can last for only a few minutes or up to several hours. Many people say that pain caused by a heart attack is the worst they have ever experienced.

Other symptoms of heart attack are anxiety, nausea, vomiting, sweating, shortness of breath, dizziness, weakness, and (very rarely) loss of consciousness. Remember, these are the usual symptoms of heart attack. In as many as 15 percent of all heart attacks, patients experience no pain or other symptoms. Doctors use a variety of techniques to determine whether a patient has had a heart attack.

Physical Examination

Sometimes the doctor, using a stethoscope, can hear certain heart sounds that are suggestive of heart attack. A whooshing sound indicates a heart murmur. Although people with normal, healthy hearts may have slight murmurs, abnormal murmurs may indicate that damage has been done by a heart attack.

The damaged heart may also make a galloping sound, so called because the cadence resembles a horse's gallop.

Electrocardiogram

Between 80 and 85 percent of all heart attacks can be detected by an electrocardiogram (EKG), a device that measures the electrical currents generated by the heart. The EKG works by picking up the very tiny currents occurring at each beat of the heart, amplifying the beats through the electrocardiograph machine, and then translating the results onto a graphic record. From the graph, the doctor can tell what the heart rate is and if the rhythm is normally paced. If an abnormality is found, the location of the problem can also be detected through the EKG graph. An EKG takes about ten minutes, is completely safe, and is not painful. All you feel is the suction of electrode cups placed on your chest.

Blood Tests

Those heart attacks undetectable by an EKG may be confirmed through blood tests. An elevated white blood cell count is one indication of heart attack. Another is an increase in the level of certain enzymes in the blood. When the heart muscle is injured by a heart attack, it releases into the blood the CPK, SGOT, and LDH enzymes. For example, CPK usually starts to increase within 12 hours after a heart attack and usually returns to normal within 48 hours. By measuring the blood's enzyme content for several days, physicians may learn more about the heart attack and make a rough estimate of when it occurred. One of the problems with using blood tests to confirm a heart attack is that it can take up to 48 hours to get the results.

Body Temperature

Your body temperature usually rises to 100°F during a heart attack. Of course, there are many reasons for an elevated body temperature, so it's not a particularly valuable diagnostic tool.

Other Tests

Heart attacks may be determined by tests that are more complicated than those just described. These include the thallium test, which uses radioactive isotopes, and cardiac catheterization, which provides physicians with moving X-rays of the heart and arteries.

EARLY TREATMENT

Immediately after your heart attack you will probably be given one or more of the following medications and treatments. Most will be discontinued after the early days of recovery.

- **Oxygen.** Since part of the heart has suffered from a lack of oxygen, most doctors believe that giving oxygen via a face mask can be beneficial.
- **Morphine.** Sometimes the pain and discomfort associated with a heart attack can be quite severe. Narcotics, most commonly morphine, help relieve this pain.
- **Diuretics.** When the injured heart is not pumping normally, fluid buildup, called *congestion,* can occur in other organs. Diuretics, which make a patient urinate more frequently, relieve this congestion.
- **Vasodilators.** These drugs are used to relieve congestion and lessen the heart's workload. They expand the arteries, thus facilitating blood flow to body parts that

may be suffering from a lack of oxygen. Nitrates, especially nitroglycerin, are the vasodilators most often prescribed.

- **Antiarrhythmic agents.** A heart attack may cause the heart to develop "electrical" problems. As a result, the heart may be pumping too fast, too slowly, or out of sequence. Antiarrhythmic drugs are used to correct such problems. Quinidine is the most popular anti-arrhythmic.

- **Surgery.** If the patient is in the hospital an hour or two after the onset of the heart attack, it may be possible to operate on the heart. Bypass surgery, involving redirection of blood around the blocked artery, may be performed. Another option is angioplasty, which involves widening the coronary artery by inserting a small balloon at the point of blockage. And then there is infusion of tissue plasminogen actuator (TPA), streptokinase, or a similar enzyme into the coronary artery. This treatment dissolves the blockage or clot that is obstructing blood flow. (See chapter 5 for a detailed discussion of these surgical procedures.)

THE HEALING PROCESS

Never underestimate the healing ability of your heart. It is a very tough organ, and it can withstand a lot of damage, provided it has enough time to heal.

A few days after a heart attack, the heart will begin to heal itself, but the repairs will not be complete for about six weeks. During this time the damaged area of the heart forms a very tough scar tissue. At the same time, other coronary arteries open tiny new branches and begin to deliver blood to the weakened area of muscle. This phenomenon is called *collateral circulation*.

In almost all instances, the heart can heal completely. If your heart has been very badly damaged, you may need surgery or drugs to help in your recovery process. Do not be alarmed if that proves to be the case for you. Many people live full, active lives with the aid of medication or surgical intervention.

During recovery, physical and emotional rest are crucial for the heart attack patient. At first you may need assistance with even the simplest tasks, such as feeding, bathing, shaving, and getting out of bed, but you must understand that these are special measures designed to help you get past the initial days of recovery. Don't resist them. You'll soon have your independence. In fact, the recovery process can be quite rapid; some patients progress from complete bedrest to sitting and then walking in days. Exactly when you actually get back on your feet depends on your doctor's judgment, the extent of your heart injury, the rate of healing, and whether or not you have developed complications.

Returning to the more strenuous activities of daily life is an individual matter, too. Most patients can expect to resume their normal activities within a month or two. Later chapters of this book will discuss in detail the convalescence (chapter 9) and the conditioning (chapter 14) phases of recovery.

One thing is true of every recovering heart patient: No matter how badly your heart has been damaged, it can be healed. And you *can* recover.

3

Conditions Related to Heart Attacks

As I'm sure you have already gathered, recovering from a heart attack is an educational experience. There is so much to learn: how your body works, what a heart attack does to it, and how the body heals. In fact, there's even more to learn than you think. In addition to heart attack itself some important related conditions often occur in conjunction with the heart attack or during the recovery period. Most patients suffer from at least one of these conditions at some time. If you are one, there is no cause for alarm, but you should know something about each condition before you proceed with your convalescence.

ANGINA

Angina is a pain in the chest. It is similar to the pain of a heart attack, but while the pain of a heart attack often lasts several hours, the pain of angina will usually subside after several minutes.

Angina is the heart's way of telling you it is not getting enough oxygen. If any of your coronary arteries is narrowed by atherosclerosis, it is difficult for the heart to receive enough oxygenated blood while it works at a normal rate. If you make the heart work harder by exercising, getting excited, or eating a large meal, for example, it may need more oxygenated blood than can be supplied by the artery. The result is the acute discomfort you feel during an angina attack.

Angina can also cause feelings of pressure, tightness, or a tingling sensation in the chest or aches and pains in the arm. In some instances victims may have pain in their jaw, teeth, earlobe, neck, or in the area between the shoulders. Some even begin choking. The pain may be localized, or it may start in one spot and spread to others.

Angina is a warning that a coronary artery is becoming critically narrowed by atherosclerosis. Once the obstruction is complete, a heart attack will occur. Most heart attacks (80 to 90 percent) are preceded by angina, but occasionally an angina attack will follow a heart attack. When that happens, it may be an indication that another coronary artery is in danger of closing.

If you suspect that you've had an angina attack, discuss it with your doctor. (Don't fool yourself into denying that the attack has actually happened.) These pains may be the result of simple indigestion or tension in the chest-wall muscles (both of which are very common and have nothing to do with your heart), but you may also be in serious danger of having another heart attack. Your doctor will want to examine you further, probably by means of an EKG and a stress test. Some physicians automatically schedule cardiac catheterization after angina, but in my opinion, in most cases it is too radical a procedure at this stage.

The discomfort of angina usually goes away, at least temporarily, if you stop the activity that caused it. If you experience angina while walking, sit down and rest until the pain stops. Then call your doctor just to be safe. If these attacks are repeated, your doctor will probably prescribe nitroglycerin.

PULMONARY EMBOLISM

If your doctor says you have a *pulmonary embolus,* he means that a blood clot is obstructing a blood vessel in or near one of your lungs. A pulmonary embolus is caused primarily by prolonged bed rest; if you remain in bed for several days, blood can pool in your legs or pelvic area, and this pooled blood may lead to the formation of a clot. If a clot breaks off into the bloodstream, it may be carried along the major veins all the way back through the heart and into the small blood vessels of the lungs. Then the lungs become damaged because vessels supplying them with oxygenated blood and other nutrients are blocked by the embolism, causing pain or shortness of breath. The heart's right ventricle may become enlarged and begin to fail because it's not getting enough oyxgen.

In order to prevent pulmonary embolism, your doctor will want you out of bed as quickly as possible after a heart attack. If you are overweight, you may be cautioned to watch your weight, since obesity causes your circulation to get sluggish and may cause blood clots to form.

Surgery is occasionally recommended to remove blood clots, but most physicians prescribe medications. These drugs do not dissolve clots, but they do prevent others from forming. Most patients begin by taking heparin, either intravenously or by injection. However, once the heparin takes hold, most patients are switched to tablets of warfarin sodium (also known as *coumadin*). Your doctor will tell you how long you must take your medication after you've been discharged from the hospital.

Because the amount of coumadin you are taking must be precisely regulated, you may have to make several visits to your doctor's office. Taking too much of an anticlotting drug can cause serious bleeding at even the slightest provocation. If you get a small cut or nick while shaving, for example, it may be hard to stop the blood flow.

Other drugs can markedly increase coumadin's anticlotting action, and that can be harmful, even fatal. *Always tell your doctor about any over-the-counter or prescription drugs you are taking, no matter how harmless they appear to be.* Be particularly careful about aspirin, which slows the rate at which blood clots, and avoid ibuprofen products (for example, Motrin, Nuprin, Medipren, and Advil), since these drugs have aspirinlike properties. If you have to treat a headache, use only acetominophen products (for example, Tylenol, Panadol, Datril, Luquiprin), since they do not have a dangerous effect on anticlotting medication.

ARRHYTHMIAS

Your heart's "electrical wiring system" is designed to make sure that its four chambers beat in sequence. It can also increase or slow down the heartbeat during various activities. When you have a heart attack, some of the heart muscle is injured, possibly affecting an electrical pathway. As a result, the normal beating rhythm of the heart may become too fast, too slow, or irregular. These rhythm changes are called *arrhythmias*.

But even if the electrical wiring system is not damaged, arrhythmia may occur after heart attack. The attack may have irritated part of the heart muscle, causing extra or "premature" beats. These extra beats also tend to make the heart rhythm irregular.

You should now be able to understand why electrical monitoring systems (electrocardiograms) are frequently used during the first few days in the cardiac care unit. Doctors rely on these to report any rhythm changes that may have occurred after the heart attack. A patient in the cardiac care unit is monitored around the clock.

If rhythm changes are detected during the first few days in cardiac care, medications are given to correct the problem while the injured area heals or becomes less irritable. If these irregular heartbeats continue for the first few days after a heart attack, you may need to take medication for an extended period of time, even after going home. Digitalis is the oldest known drug used to treat arrhythmia. It works by delaying electrical transmissions in the heart, slowing down and steadying the heart rate. However, the disadvantage of digitalis (and other antiarrhythmic drugs) is that when taken in excess, it too may throw off the heart's natural rhythm. Make sure your doctor thoroughly explains to you the nature of your arrhythmia and your precise treatment plan.

CONGESTIVE HEART FAILURE

In addition to having an electrical system in your heart, you have an elaborate pumping system. When these pumps do not do their job, *congestive heart failure* may occur. Congestive heart failure often accompanies a heart attack, but there are other times it can happen as well.

The chain of events leading to congestive heart failure is not difficult to understand. If, for example, the heart muscle surrounding the left ventricle is severely damaged by the heart attack, this chamber will be unable to empty all the blood pumped into it. As a result, blood will begin to accumulate and wash backward, through the left atrium and the pulmonary vein. The lungs will become congested with fluid, making it difficult for you to breathe. This congestion usually shows up on a chest X-ray and can be heard by listening to the lungs with a stethoscope.

From the lungs, the congestion may go backward still farther, through the pulmonary artery, right ventricle, right atrium, and back into major veins of the body. Fluid may then collect in other body parts, such as the liver or the extremities. Some people with congestion notice swelling in their ankles and feet, particularly at the end of the day, when their shoes begin to feel too small. Others notice that their rings feel uncomfortably tight, their legs and arms become clammy, and they are overtaken by a feeling of dizziness and disorientation. When blood flows backward, not enough freshly oxygenated blood goes to the brain, limbs, and other parts of the body.

Congestive heart failure causes the kidneys to retain fluids, and as a result, you often gain weight. This is why heart patients are weighed every day in the hospital. If you find yourself gaining two to three pounds in one day, it is probably due to fluid retention. Note that gaining three pounds in a day would have to mean that you are eating more than ten times the amount that you normally eat—an almost impossible task even for the most avid gourmand.

If you have had problems with heart failure in the hospital, or suspect you may have problems during recovery at home, it's a good idea to keep a daily record of your weight during the first few weeks after your heart attack. Always weigh yourself first thing in the morning. And since excessive salt increases fluid retention, try cutting back on the amount of sodium in your diet (see chapter 12).

Drugs such as digoxin may be used to increase the pumping strength of the heart muscle, and diuretics may be prescribed to help you lose the excess fluid your body has collected. The earlier the signs of congestive heart failure are recognized and treated, the better off you will be. If you experience such symptoms, especially shortness of breath or swelling of the ankles, alert your doctor immediately.

PERICARDITIS

The heart is surrounded and protected by a sac called the *pericardium*. Under normal conditions, there is a small amount of fluid in the pericardial sac, and the heart moves easily within it. But if the sac becomes inflamed after a heart attack, pericarditis occurs. Pericarditis does no permanent damage to your heart muscle. All that has happened is that the sac surrounding your heart became irritated. A doctor listening to your heart with a stethoscope can often hear a rub or squeak that confirms the condition.

If you should develop pericarditis, you may notice discomfort in your chest, shoulders, and neck. The pain, which can vary from mild soreness to severe distress, is usually relieved by sitting up and leaning forward. You will also feel more comfortable lying down in bed.

Aspirin or indomethacin and cortisonelike drugs may be prescribed to help control the pain of pericarditis. The discomfort should disappear in a few days, but you may need to continue your medication for several weeks to make certain the problem does not recur. If pericarditis continues for longer than a month, it may be caused by more than your heart attack. Further tests will be necessary.

SILENT ISCHEMIA

Ischemia is an oxygen insufficiency of the coronary arteries that stops just short of a heart attack. If you have a narrowing in your coronary artery, you will probably experience pain. You would then sit down and rest, at which time the oxygen insufficiency would go away, and so would the pain. The pain you experience in this situation is angina; the oxygen insufficiency is ischemia.

Some people experience the insufficiency without the pain: silent ischemia. The only way you can actually know if you're having silent ischemia is by being hooked up to an EKG or to a special ambulatory monitor, which is becoming more common. The monitor, which gives the same information as an EKG, may be worn at home or at the office.

MITRAL VALVE PROLAPSE

Back in the olden days, women used to be stricken with attacks of what were quaintly called "vapors"—shortness of breath, faintness, mild palpitations. Ten years ago we began to call the ailment by a different, less romantic name: *mitral valve prolapse*.

Caused by a mild degeneration of the mitral valve, one of the four valves of the heart, mitral valve prolapse runs in families and shows up in 12 percent of all women over twenty years old. It is a very minor condition, usually treated with antibiotics for two or three days when you have dental work done. It is not life-threatening.

There is no relationship between coronary artery disease and mitral valve prolapse, but I include it here because many people have landed in the hospital emergency room complaining of faintness, dizziness, chest pains, and palpitations. Fortunately for them, what they thought was a heart attack turned out to be "the vapors"—mitral valve prolapse.

4
Your Hospital Stay

There are hospitals and hospitals. Some are huge and magnificently endowed; others are tiny, virtually mom-and-pop operations. No matter what the size is, though, nearly every hospital in the world has designated a separate section where patients can be closely monitored. Until the mid-1970s this section was usually called the intensive care unit—the ICU.

It did not take health care professionals long to notice that most of their customers in ICU were heart patients, so quite sensibly they began to subdivide many ICUs, giving those who needed heart care their own "neighborhood," which they called the cardiac care unit, or CCU. Since then intensive care has become more specialized all the time, with sections for children, for postsurgical patients, for gynecology. At one hospital I know well there are at least twelve intensive care units, including four separate cardiac care units. Of course, all hospitals are not alike, but they do have many things in common, especially when it comes to intensive care.

THE CARDIAC CARE UNIT

Stepping into the cardiac care unit (CCU) of any major hospital is a little like entering another world. Vast networks of tubes, catheters, and electrical wires intertwine like mini-superhighways across each patient's bed. Video monitors abound, flashing green or yellow lights. And all around, green-, blue-, or white-suited men and women move briskly from room to room. You can't tell whether it's day or night. In the world of the CCU, the lights are always on.

The CCU is not a comforting place in the traditional sense—it's no wonder that most people feel uneasy in these strange surroundings—but for the patient with a heart condition, there is no better place to be. Here you are closely monitored by computerized equipment, which can detect and report the slightest changes in your heart rate or blood pressure, and you are cared for by some of the most competent medical professionals in the entire hospital.

Most CCUs are set up so that you receive "primary care," which means that the nurse-to-patient ratio is one to one (compared to the one-to-eight nurse-to-patient ratio of most other hospital floors). Cardiac nurses may have special training in heart patient care and emergency treatment.

Not everyone in a CCU has had a heart attack. Patients are admitted there for a variety of reasons, sometimes just for testing and observation. For instance, if physicians cannot obtain accurate heart rhythm readings through electrocardiogram testing (it is estimated that 15 percent of all patients cannot be diagnosed by an EKG), they may send their patients to the CCU for enzyme tests or cardiac catheterization. In this way they can help prove their diagnoses and at the same time prevent complications from developing.

Should someone experience cardiac arrest in the unit, a special code is announced over the hospital's public address system. Different hospitals use different codes for cardiac arrest—"Dr. Heart," "Code Blue," "Dr. C.R.," and "Code 999" are examples—but all alert the heart team to action.

Most patients and families who witness an emergency are astonished by the team's precision and swiftness. True, witnessing such an experience may be somewhat upsetting, but it is dramatic proof that CCU patients are well served.

In fact, patients in the CCU have relatively few complaints. One of the most common ones voiced by CCU patients is that the lights are always kept on. I once had a patient ask to see me in the middle of the night. When I got to his bedside, he seemed almost embarrassed. "Look, I didn't mind the catheterization, and I'm not complaining about all these tubes I have in my arm. But I just can't sleep with the lights on," he said plaintively.

One story that made the rounds was about a seventy-year-old patient who left his bed and climbed into bed with another patient who happened to be a seventy-year-old woman. Fortunately the woman was heavily sedated, so she didn't even notice that she had company. The nurse noticed, though, and when she asked the man why he was playing musical beds, he gave her a straightforward answer: "The light over my bed is too bright; I came in here where it wouldn't be shining in my eyes."

In addition to the constant light, the frequent interruptions of the CCU staff can be disorienting as well. While it is reassuring for patients to know that staff members are watching them 24 hours a day, carefully observing their progress, it can make it difficult to get much sleep. However, once you leave the CCU, your sleep patterns should return to normal.

TYPICAL CCU PROCEDURES

Most of the machines in the CCU are used to monitor your vital signs. You will probably be connected to an EKG, which keeps track of the electrical currents generated by the heart. The connection is made by two flat electrodes or tiny suction cups that stick to various spots on your chest. There is no pain involved in this procedure. All you feel is the lubricating jelly that is spread over your chest area to ensure better suction.

Additionally, you will probably be connected to quite a bit of tubing, including intravenous tubes, a nasogastric tube, a chest tube, and a catheter. The intravenous tubing allows for *intravenous* ("through the vein") feeding and prompt administration of medicine if it is necessary. The chest tube, which emits a constant gurgling sound, is used to remove air or fluid that might have accumulated around the heart. The catheter, which is inserted in your bladder, is used to monitor your urine output and determine whether your kidneys are functioning properly.

Finally, you will be given low doses of oxygen through a special nasal tube or a mask; this helps to lessen the heart's workload during recovery. And various other tubes or catheters may be inserted in your arteries and veins in order to measure the heart's performance throughout the day.

Physicians and nurses will come by to check your progress quite regularly. This may seem like a nuisance, since they will often have to wake you up to check on you, but try to cooperate. These checks are being done for your own good, and besides, they don't take all that long. Maybe it will help you to know exactly what the nurses or doctors are checking for during these brief examinations. Using a stethoscope, they check for normal heart sounds, that may have changed a bit after your heart attack, indicating a potential problem. This same stethoscope may be used to listen to your lungs, since congestion often begins in this area, and excess water in the lower portion of your lungs can be heard. During these exams you may be asked to pronounce the words "ninety-nine" or some other deeply resonant sound that requires the use of your full lung capacity.

The nurses or doctors will check for congestion. Because congestion can cause water buildup in the ankles or at the base of the spine, the examiner will press on the skin's surface in these spots. If an indentation remains, your body could be flooding with congestive fluid, which is a sign that diuretics should be prescribed.

You may be asked how many pillows you are using to sleep. This may sound like a strange question, but it's perfectly sensible, and the answer is important. If you require more than two pillows to lie down comfortably, your lungs may be congested—a potentially dangerous situation that must be checked out immediately. (It could mean congestive heart failure.) The examiner will listen for fluid in your lungs, check your veins to see if they're distended, and feel your ankles and the bottom of your spine.

Be prepared, too, for regular blood pressure checks, blood tests, and requests for urine samples. There will probably be times when you feel as if you're being invaded from all sides, but have patience. All of these tests assist the medical staff in measuring your progress during this critical time.

A typical stay in the CCU is only a few days. If there are complications, such as heart failure, arrhythmias, angina, or pulmonary embolism, it may be somewhat longer. Toward the end of your time in the CCU, you will be encouraged to start moving around at least a little, by dangling your legs from the bed, shaving yourself, brushing your hair, feeding yourself, or using the bedside commode. The last day in CCU is often spent learning about recovery and focusing on the healing process.

THE STEP-DOWN UNIT

During most of the time you spend in the CCU you're exhausted, disoriented, and possibly a little frightened. You're probably under heavy sedation, and much of the time you really don't know what is going on. If all goes well, after about 48 hours you will move into what's called the step-down unit. Separate from the CCU, the step-down unit is rather like the departure lounge at the airport. Think of it as one step closer to home.

In the step-down unit there is still some monitoring of blood pressure, heart rate, and other vital signs, but the nurse-to-patient ratio decreases, since patients do not require constant supervision. You will be much more active here than you were in the CCU. In most instances you will be encouraged to take short walks around the unit. A radio-operated monitor will keep track of your heart rate during these brief strolls.

Logic would suggest that a patient should be relieved and happy to graduate to the step-down unit, but it's not always quite so simple as that. For many people, the step-down unit represents a return to reality. The initial scare is over, and the morphine has worn off. If you're a smoker, you're probably going through nicotine withdrawal. Now the worrying can really begin. "Am I going to die?" is replaced by more mundane concerns: "How am I going to pay for this?" or "What if I lose my job?" or "I'm supposed to make a casserole for a party this weekend."

Anxiety or depression in the step-down unit are to be expected. If you find yourself feeling this way, try using your time productively. Now is a good time to get your cardiac life in order. If you'd like to talk to the dietitian about how to change your diet when you get home, ask your doctor to arrange it. Learn about your medication. Start thinking about formal cardiac rehabilitation, the program that will guide you through your recovery in the months to come. Talk to the doctors and nurses, and ask to see the staff social worker. With luck these distractions will keep you from worrying about the sales conference you're about to miss.

There was a time when most heart attack patients spent about six weeks in the hospital, but today, provided there are no extra complications, the average hospital stay after a heart attack is less than a week. One reason is that patients tend to recover faster in the privacy and comfort of home. Another is that doctors and hospital administrators know that insurance providers may not reimburse them for the days a patient is kept in the hospital beyond a week if there are no other complications.

Keep in mind that there are no rules when it comes to the length of a hospital stay; each case is different. Some patients may need to stay longer for extra testing. Others may go home and then be readmitted for diagnostic or other procedures, such as heart catheterization or a stress test. I schedule my patients for cardiac catheterization and/or a mini–stress test before they go home. If you are concerned about the length of your hospital stay, discuss it with your doctor. He or she should explain the factors that determine the duration of your hospitalization. If you aren't satisfied with the explanation, ask to talk to a hospital social worker or patient advocate.

VISITORS

Visitors to the CCU react in many different ways. Some cry, partly out of relief at seeing their loved one alive and partly out of shock at the amount of machinery surrounding the beds. Some people faint; others become almost manic, laughing loudly at inappropriate moments. Silly arguments, about where the teenaged daughter is going to go to college or who should have picked up the laundry, are commonplace, as are other domestic squabbles.

Suffice it to say that during the crisis of a heart attack, the family dynamics are usually tremendously disrupted. It is only normal for your family to act a bit out of character the first time they see you in the CCU. They, too, need time to adjust to the reality of your illness and the events ahead. It is important for your family to understand that the CCU is your starting point on the road back to health. All those monitors, wires, and tubes surrounding you are designed not to signal your death but to help you get better. If nothing else, you should assure your family that while you may feel tired and a little weak, you aren't in pain.

Part of a doctor's and a nurse's job is to spend time with family members. In fact, as far as I'm concerned, it's one of the most important parts of a doctor's job. If your doctor won't take the time to educate and sympathize with your family, perhaps you should think about getting another doctor. Encourage your loved ones to ask your doctor questions and to speak openly about their anxiety during this critical time. A trained social worker who has special expertise in cardiac care may also be available for consultation. If no one comes forward to talk to you and your family at this time, ask for an appointment. These conversations should take place very early in the recovery period, before unwarranted fears and misconceptions are allowed to take root.

When you do have your talk, don't be afraid to bring up your concerns about money. Social workers are there to help you and your family with financial concerns. They will try to answer your questions and, if necessary, refer you to a financial counselor at the hospital. Social workers also know about community resources available for recovering heart patients and their families. They can be instrumental in connecting you with the support groups, cardiac rehabilitation programs, or even legal assistance you may need when you leave the hospital.

Hospital volunteers assigned specifically to the cardiac care unit are another valuable resource for heart patients. Most of these individuals have suffered a heart attack or have helped a loved one through recovery. They speak from experience, which is something you and your family may really appreciate right now.

Of course, no matter how upset your family may be, they must adhere strictly to the rules of the hospital when they visit you in the CCU. Some of the rules may seem strict (for instance, allowing only two guests at a time in the room), but they are designed for the well-being of you and the other patients. There may be certain restrictions on flowers, gifts (especially food), and television viewing that visitors should know about. Naturally, there's no smoking allowed in the CCU. Many of the patients in CCU use oxygen, which is extremely inflammable if exposed to the open flame of a cigarette or lighter.

The staff of any CCU will have dozens of stories about visitors who tried to smuggle in contraband to recovering patients. I've seen candy, ice cream, cakes, cartons of cigarettes, even a case of twelve-year-old Scotch. I've seen caterers try to make their way into the CCU with cans of Sterno. One day a CCU nurse looked up to see a woman on her way in to visit her husband. The nurse was admiring the coat the woman was wearing, and then she noticed a peculiar bulge in the front. Not enjoying her role as prison warden but knowing that her job was to protect her patient, the nurse moved closer to have a look. The woman had bought her husband something to cheer him up: an eight-week-old puppy.

GETTING YOU UP AND MOVING

Before the mid-1960s, heart patients spent four to six weeks flat on their backs in a hospital bed. Even getting up to use the toilet was forbidden. Now we know, among many other things, that too much bed rest is bad for the circulation and may even cause pulmonary embolism. As soon as possible, you will be encouraged to start your circulation flowing normally again. Even during the first few days of your recovery you'll be making small but progressive movements.

Your first activity will probably be dangling your feet over the side of the bed. Soon afterward you will progress to the bathroom, where you will take a shower, either sitting or standing. Eventually you will begin walking up and down the hospital corridor (a sure sign that you will soon be going home). There are gentle leg and arm exercises for improving muscle tone and joint mobility.

At first you may feel weak when you try to get up, but the weakness is probably due more to inactivity than to your heart's condition. (Astronauts have the same "deconditioning" effect after being weightless for some time.) You'll get stronger as you increase your daily activities.

Do not be afraid that you are doing too much. Remember, you are in the safest place possible after a heart attack, with doctors and nurses monitoring your activities and looking out for your welfare. However, should you honestly think something is wrong—for instance, if you have chest pains, dizziness, severe headaches, or blood in your urine or stool—tell the medical staff immediately.

CARDIAC FUNCTION TESTS

Before you walk out the hospital door, you will most likely undergo a number of tests to ensure that you are ready for discharge. Let's take a quick look at each of them.

The Mini–Stress Test

The mini–stress test enables physicians to monitor the heart's functions when it is working. The test is quite accurate. You will be asked to ride a stationary bicycle or to walk on a treadmill, both of which can be adjusted for speed, and you will be pushed until your heartbeat goes up to about 120 beats per minute.

Don't confuse this mini–stress test with the full stress test. A mini–stress test is done only after a heart attack, usually the day before you are discharged. A full stress test is not administered until your heart has healed, at least six weeks after a heart attack.

In the mini–stress test, painless electrodes are attached to your chest for monitoring purposes. The speed of the treadmill or bicycle is increased until your heart rate is about 120 beats per minute. Since this is about the maximum rate at which your heart beats for many activities at home, physicians can project at this point how your heart will perform during normal daily life. They can determine what restrictions, if any, you should have during your first days at home.

The mini–stress test will take about 30 minutes, although you will actually ride the bike or walk on the treadmill for no more than 12 minutes. Remember, a mini–stress test is not an endurance test. Should you begin to overexert yourself, the procedure will be stopped.

As a rule, patients who do well in a mini–stress test will do very well during the first year after their heart attack. The current statistics show that you will have 98 percent chance of not dying from a heart attack in the coming year if you do well on your predischarge stress test. If you do badly on the mini–stress test, you probably won't be allowed to go home. Further tests will be prescribed. Most patients who do poorly on the mini–stress test will be given a cardiac catheterization.

The Full Stress Test

The most usual of the stress tests is the full stress test, which is not usually performed until six weeks after a heart attack. During the full stress test the patient is exercised quite vigorously—normally on a treadmill—and his heart rate is measured. (Heart rates of 150 to 170 beats per minute are quite common.) The full stress test is not quite so accurate as a thallium stress test, but it costs considerably less.

Thallium Stress Test

In a thallium stress test, also called a *thallium scan*, radioactive chemicals are injected into the bloodstream and their movement is traced by a special camera that detects any insufficiency or blockage in the coronary arteries. (By the way, don't be frightened by the word *radioactive*. The material that is used contains less radiation than an X-ray.) Your physician will look at how the chemicals are handled by the heart. Should these chemicals not flow smoothly in and out of the heart's muscle, certain areas of your heart may have been damaged and need repair.

If a twenty-five-year-old woman came to see me complaining of chest pains, I might recommend an ordinary stress test. If a sixty-year-old man came in with the same type of pain, I would probably schedule him for a thallium stress test, since I wouldn't believe the treadmill test if the results were negative. Whereas the stress test is accurate about 85 percent of the time, the thallium test is 98 percent accurate. Unfortunately the cost for this kind of accuracy is not low; the thallium test costs about $1,000.

The Technesium Scan

Another chemical that may be injected into the bloodstream is technesium. A technesium scan enables the doctors to determine how the walls of the heart are working and how much blood the ventricles of the heart are ejecting on each beat. Doctors are interested in this because it indicates whether the function of the heart is improving or getting worse.

Ambulatory and Other Monitors

Another test requires the patient to wear the Holter, a 24-hour ambulatory EKG monitor. This device determines the heart's response to everyday activities and can detect arrhythmias. If you undergo this procedure, you will be requested to keep a detailed written account of the day's activities while wearing the Holter so that your heart's reactions to various activities can be properly assessed.

Since the early 1980s, heart patients, usually high-risk patients or ones with artificial pacemakers, have been able to take a variation of the Holter monitor home from the hospital with them. One example is the transtelephonic monitor, which enables a patient to transmit EKG readings to a doctor or cardiac rehabilitation center over the phone. Patients may be asked to "phone in" their EKG reading as many as three times a day.

The only drawback to the monitors that are now being used is that in order to take full advantage of them, patients have to know something is wrong. With a newly developed entry into the field of electronic ambulatory monitors—Heart Guard—that will no longer be the case. Heart Guard, which works by means of electrodes attached to the chest, will constantly monitor the heart and feed the information to a "central office." When something goes wrong with your heart, even if you don't feel a thing, the information is recorded and passed along immediately to your doctor's office by means of computer linking. In patients who are unstable or who have many chronic health problems, electronic ambulatory monitors are invaluable. Heart Guard is a virtual lifeline for the heart patient.

Cardiac Catheterization

For assessing the heart's condition, the best diagnostic procedure around is cardiac catheterization. Nothing else short of open heart surgery can provide your physician with a clearer, more detailed view of the way your heart functions and the trouble spots that may need repair.

Cardiac catheterization is usually recommended after other tests (the EKG, the stress test, the thallium stress test, or the technesium scan) have indicated that there is a potential problem with your heart. Sometimes this procedure is done on an emergency basis, when your heart attack has been very severe or if you are in danger of having another attack very soon. Everyone undergoes cardiac catheterization before surgery, but only about half of all patients who are catheterized go on to have surgery.

You must be hospitalized for cardiac catheterization, but most patients leave the hospital 24 to 36 hours after the procedure has been completed. Because cardiac catheterization must be done in a completely sterile environment, you are draped and covered, just as if you are having an operation. The doctors, nurses, and technicians wear the same gowns and gloves they wear in the operating room.

Cardiac catheterization takes about an hour and is done under local anesthetic; you are awake throughout the procedure. It begins when a polyurethane tube is inserted into an artery or vein in the groin area or the crease of the elbow. If the catheter is inserted in a vein, it is advanced into the right side of the heart and into the pulmonary arteries. If the catheter is inserted in an artery, it is advanced into the aorta, threaded through the aortic valve, and ultimately inserted into the heart's left ventricle.

When the catheter reaches the heart's chamber, a special radio-opaque dye that can be seen on film is injected through the catheter and into the heart area. At this point you may feel a wave of heat, as if you were standing directly in front of a household heater. The "hot flash" does not last more than five or ten seconds. As the dye begins to circulate through the heart, the room lights are turned off, and an X-ray camera is used to film its path through the heart. Dye is injected into the three coronary arteries, and various high-speed movies are taken.

Other tests may be performed while the catheterization is going on. Delicate sensors in the tip of or connected to the catheter can measure the volume of blood pumped by the heart and show if this flow is less than normal, or the catheter may be used to measure the electrical activity of your heart. Blood samples drawn through the catheter may be measured for oxygen content.

You should not feel any pain after the catheterization. The small black-and-blue mark or lump under your skin at the point of the insertion of the catheter should disappear in about a week.

Your physician will use the catheterization results as a "road map" of your heart. Sometimes this map will reveal that there is no further heart problem at all. At other times the map will reveal where trouble exists and help physicians determine the treatment that will best handle the problem.

HURRY UP AND WAIT

My next-door neighbor, not a patient of mine, had a heart attack. I went to see him a few days after he came home from the hospital and asked how he was feeling and how his hospital stay had been. What he told me was something I hear at least once a week from one of my own patients. He said that the heart attack hadn't been so bad, and he didn't even mind the food or being awakened at all hours. What almost drove him crazy, he said, was having to wait for what seemed like weeks to get the results of his tests.

He was exaggerating, of course, but he was right about one thing. One of the most frustrating aspects of being a heart patient is having to wait for test results. Naturally you want to know the results immediately, since only they can tell you how much progress you are making, but there's no such thing as "immediately" when it comes to test results. When you are in the CCU, tests are being run hourly, but once you get out into the world of step-down and beyond, you have to wait your turn with everyone else. And like everyone else you'll be exposed to delays, in the laboratory, the radiology department, or other diagnostic sections of the hospital.

Since there is nothing you can do about these delays, try to be patient. And while you are waiting, remind yourself that "no news is good news."

OVERTESTING

Some patients feel as if they're being overtested. They begin to wonder whether so many diagnostic procedures are really necessary. If you have such concerns, discuss them with your doctor. It's important that you understand the doctor's strategy for diagnosis and plans for helping you to get better. The more you know about what all those beeping, buzzing, blinking machines provided for modern heart care can do, the more confidence you can have in the doctor who prescribes them.

5

Surgery and Other Cardiac Procedures

At some time in your treatment, you will probably have a long and serious discussion with your family and your physician concerning the possibility of bypass surgery, angioplasty, pacemaker implantation, or some other sophisticated heart procedure. Surgery is not an easy subject to talk about at any time, let alone right after you've had a heart attack, but I'm afraid the discussion is inevitable.

Most people view a major medical intervention with apprehension, and so they should. Surgery is always a serious business. In my practice I've found that the more my patients and their families know about the procedures, the more relaxed they become about the choices that must be made. In order to become less anxious about your treatment, take the time to learn about the heart procedures that are most widely used today. The following is a brief account of many standard procedures. While you read these sections, keep in mind that thousands of people go through each one (or maybe more than one) every year. They are all proven lifesavers.

ANGIOPLASTY

A percutaneous transluminal coronary angioplasty (PCTA) is commonly known as *angioplasty,* or "balloon treatment." This procedure, which was introduced to the United States by a Swiss surgeon, Andreas Gruentzig, in 1977, is usually performed in large, well-equipped medical centers, and for many heart patients it has become a preferable alternative to surgery.

Angioplasty involves widening the inside of a narrowed coronary artery with a special catheter. However, unlike the catheter used in cardiac catheterization (described in chapter 4), this one is equipped with a small balloon on its tip. When the catheter reaches the point of blockage, the balloon is inflated, and the fatty material is pressed against the wall of the artery. When the balloon is deflated, the fat remains compressed, and blood flows freely through the artery.

Angioplasties are usually performed in the cardiac catheterization laboratory, and you are anesthetized (in the arm or groin), draped, and covered much like the patient who is undergoing cardiac catheterization. This form of treatment for coronary artery disease has become increasingly popular, as more and more doctors are becoming proficient at it. In some medical centers it is done as often as open heart surgery, and the number of angioplasties performed throughout the country is expected to increase dramatically within the next few years.

However, many cardiologists, myself included, remain somewhat skeptical about angioplasty. The procedure is still relatively new, and its success is by no means guaranteed; in a very small percentage of patients, arteries have been found to close again just minutes after the balloon has been removed. Many patients require repeat angioplasties, time and time again on the same coronary artery. It is not at all uncommon for patients to need an angioplasty every six months. For them it is considerably less time-consuming and more economical to have bypass surgery.

THROMBOLYSIS

In addition to angioplasty, there is another new, increasingly popular heart procedure, called *thrombolysis.* During this process, streptokinase or a related drug called *tissue plaminogen activator* (TPA) is used to dissolve fresh blood clots. This procedure is prescribed only under very special circumstances. If a patient is brought to the hospital during the onset of a life-threatening heart attack, the drugs are infused, again through a catheter in the arm or groin, to destroy the obstructing clot. The whole procedure takes about 20 minutes.

Thrombolysis is not for everyone. First, you must be in the midst of a heart attack for it to be effective (yet another reason to get to the hospital as quickly after a heart attack as possible). Second, the procedure does nothing to solve the problem of atherosclerosis, which probably caused the clot in the first place. Therefore, after thrombolysis you are still left with narrowed arteries, which could cause problems in the future. Third, if you have stomach problems, especially a gastric or duodenal ulcer, you may begin to bleed uncontrollably.

All in all, thrombolysis is an important emergency procedure, but very often it's only the first step in your treatment. It is quite possible that after thrombolysis you will need angioplasty or bypass surgery.

BYPASS SURGERY

Since the early 1970s, *bypass surgery* has been the mainstay of treatment for advanced coronary artery disease. In fact, if you are about to undergo or have just undergone bypass surgery, you are probably among the majority of people reading this book.

Technically known as coronary artery bypass grafting (CABG), the procedure is basically used to circumvent (or bypass) blood around a blocked artery. Traditionally, it involves removing a vein from the lower leg and grafting one of its ends into a small opening made in the aorta. The other end of the vein is sewn into an opening made below the blockage in the diseased artery, creating a new passageway for blood flow. It is like creating a detour on a crowded freeway, allowing cars to flow around a heavily congested area.

Bypass surgery can take as few as three or as many as nine hours or more, depending on the number of bypass grafts you need. (By the way, much too much has been made of the significance of the number of grafts. I once heard Henry Kissinger and Alexander Haig comparing numbers. As I recall, Kissinger said he had had four, and Haig proudly announced that he had had five, as if they were discussing golf scores!) After the operation, you are taken to the ICU or CCU, where you are closely monitored for at least 48 hours.

Many surgeons are beginning to use an alternative to the leg vein for bypass surgery. This new approach involves mobilizing the internal mammary artery in the chest wall, which is not essential to any of the body's basic functions. During the procedure, surgeons sew one end of the vessel onto a coronary artery, thereby allowing blood to flow past the blockage. Many patients prefer this new type of bypass, since it seems to work better and the leg vein procedure often leaves scars on the leg.

Cardiologists have good reason to recommend bypass surgery to so many of their patients. The latest figures reveal that you have an excellent chance of surviving the surgery, and your chances of returning to your normal activity level after the surgery, with no discomfort or pain, are also extremely high. People who have bypass surgery usually do very well, and so they should; from an anatomical viewpoint, the thing that has been causing the symptoms (angina, shortness of breath, chest pains, whatever) has been removed.

What's more, surgical advancements are being made on the bypass procedure all the time. Some of the most sophisticated medical equipment found in any medical center is used during the operation, including the remarkable heart-lung machine, which makes it possible for surgeons to empty your heart of blood while they are working on it. Your heart is temporarily put out of use during this time, available for the surgeons to do their repairs. The machine actually takes over lung and heart functions during your surgery. Unoxygenated blood from the veins, which would normally flow back into the heart, is reoxygenated by the machine and prepared for another trip through the circulatory system.

Other improvements in bypass surgery have resulted from studies that show the heart heals faster if the body is kept at a cool temperature throughout the surgery. And then there are the new surgical tools and machines, including advanced fiber-optic catheters, special monitoring equipment that keeps surgeons constantly apprised of your heart pressure while they are at work, and the cell-saver, which conserves your own blood during surgery and eliminates the need for blood transfusion.

Before the mid-1970s many doctors thought it was a mistake to perform bypass surgery on patients who were over seventy years old or very seriously ill, but the thinking now is that virtually everyone is a candidate for bypass surgery. A few months ago I saw a patient who illustrates this point perfectly. He had just had a heart attack, and a cardiac catheterization showed that two of his arteries were seriously blocked. Bypass surgery was clearly indicated. The only problem was that he had cancer of the kidneys; his doctor had told him that he had only a few years left.

Even if I had been inclined to talk him out of heart surgery, which I wasn't, he wouldn't have listened anyway. "Look, I know I'm going to be dead in two or three years," he said, "but it's going to be the cancer that kills me, not my heart. And I want to live out the years I have left with a healthy heart. I want to have the surgery." And so he did, with my blessing.

PACEMAKERS

In our discussion of arrhythmias I explained that sometimes the heart rate becomes irregular. The heartbeats are too rapid or too slow, and the result is a hindering of efficient cardiac function. This occurs when the heart's natural pacemaker is not doing its job properly. Fortunately we now have something that can take the place of the heart's natural pacemaker—a mechanical one.

Some pacemakers are only temporary. You may be fitted with a temporary pacemaker while you are resting in the cardiac care unit after surgery, for instance. These pacemakers are actually pacemaker catheters, which are inserted into a vein and then advanced up into the heart. They are usually removed within a few days, when the heart has rested enough to keep its own pace.

The pacemakers that we are accustomed to hearing about are the permanent ones. If your doctor thinks that you should have one, he'll set up a meeting between you and the thoracic surgeon who will be inserting it. During the meeting you'll find out how the device is inserted and what you can expect from wearing it. You'll also get to see one. Most patients are surprised by the size of today's pacemakers. They are not the large, bulging "packs" of yesterday; most battery packs are about the size of a pocket watch, and they have two wires, called *leads,* attached to them.

To implant the pacemaker, the surgeon makes an incision just beneath the skin in the upper chest area. Next he makes very small incisions in a vein just beneath the collarbone and threads the leads through until they enter the right side of the heart. Finally, he makes a small pocket just below the skin, places the battery pack inside, and sews up the incision. When this small incision heals, the bulge of the pacemaker is barely visible.

New advances in technology have lengthened the life of a pacemaker to anywhere from 10 to 15 years, at which time you will have to have the old one removed and a new one implanted. Before that time, however, you'll have to have periodic checks to ensure that the device is running well and using energy efficiently. With the proper equipment (for example, the transtelephonic monitors, described in chapter 4), these check-ups may be conducted by telephone.

Pacemaker wearers can expect to lead long, healthy, active lives. In fact, most of my patients find that they have more energy than they have had in a very long time. There is no reason to curtail your activities if you have a pacemaker. However, there are a few precautions that every pacemaker wearer must take:

- Carry the name and type of pacemaker you are wearing with you at all times so that medical professionals may identify your needs in an emergency. The special identification bracelets are best, but if you can't bring yourself to wear one, carry a card in your wallet or handbag that identifies your pacemaker type, your doctor's name, and the medications you are taking.
- Get in the habit of checking your pulse every day (see

page 157 for instructions). Ask your doctor about the range of your heart rate, and call him or her right away if it goes under or over these limits.

- Know the early warning signs that your pacemaker may be failing: dizziness, fainting, heart palpitations, difficulty in breathing, unexplained weight gain, and swelling of the ankles and legs. If any of these symptoms occurs, notify your doctor at once.

One thing you need not worry about any longer is the danger of the effect of electronic wave transmissions, such as those in electronic cash registers and microwave ovens, on your pacemaker. Before the mid-1970s some pacemakers were sensitive to those devices, and patients were warned not to be around them, but those pacemakers are no longer in use. With the more modern pacemakers this problem has disappeared, and the old restrictions no longer apply. If your pacemaker is very old or if you just need some reassurance that you're not in any danger, talk to your doctor.

HEART TRANSPLANTS

In 1967 South Africa's Dr. Christiaan Barnard did what was once believed impossible. He implanted a human heart in Louis Waskansky, a fifty-five-year-old man.

Today transplants are performed in medical centers across the nation. In fact, there are now close to 1,000 people in the United States alone who have had the operation. Many of these people enjoy a quality of life they never expected before undergoing the procedure; some have even been able to return to work.

Much of our recent success with heart transplants is due to cyclosporin, a drug that was not available when the procedure was first performed. Cyclosporin has proved critical in suppressing the white-cell growth that causes foreign tissue to be rejected. By using this drug, doctors have been able to reduce the frequency and severity of rejection of a transplanted heart, as well as decreasing the incidence of infection in transplant patients.

While heart transplants don't make the front pages anymore, they are by no means commonplace, and becoming a candidate for heart transplant is not an easy process. The requirements are strict and the exceptions virtually nonexistent. Transplant candidates must be under sixty years of age (until quite recently the age was fifty), free of any other illness, and at the very end stage of heart disease (meaning that the heart absolutely cannot function any longer). These criteria are changing all the time. For instance, a woman who had undergone a hysterectomy was recently approved for a transplant; six months earlier she would have been ineligible. However, the rules are unlikely to loosen up to any significant degree.

Because the operation is so special, and so relatively rare, I am reluctant to discuss in general terms what the effects of a transplant are likely to be on the health of any heart patient. I suggest that you discuss this and all other aspects of the transplant operation with your doctor.

ARTIFICIAL HEARTS AND TRANS-SPECIES TRANSPLANTS

In 1982 Dr. William DeVries implanted the world's first artificial heart, called the Jarvik-7, in patient Barney Clark. In 1984 an infant known only as Baby Fae was given a baboon heart to replace her own failing one.

The artificial heart and trans-species transplant are still both highly experimental. Barney Clark lived 112 days after his operation; Baby Fae died after only 20 days. Surgeons believe that it will take at least a decade of refinement before either of these procedures can become as effective as heart transplants. And then there is the problem of expense. Barney Clark's Jarvik-7 cost $30,000 to install and far more to maintain.

At the moment the artificial heart and trans-species transplants are being used only as stop-gap measures, in order to keep patients alive long enough to arrange for a heart transplant. As you can imagine, the patient selection is even more stringent than it is with transplants. Prospective patients for these procedures, even on a stop-gap basis, must have no other options for staying alive. They must pass an extensive screening process by a surgical selection committee. Anyone too sick or not sick enough will instantly be ruled out by the committee. So will diabetics or people with most other chronic health problems.

Right now it is best to view the artificial heart and trans-species transplants as experiments. We can only hope that these experiments will help us understand the heart more fully and give us new insights into how it can be repaired.

LASERS AND BEYOND

What are the heart treatments of the future? Right now, scientists are exploring the possibility of using *lasers,* hoping that the superfast beams of energy might be able to burn through plaque blockages in the arteries. So far, though, the energy source has proved to be so strong that along with destroying the damaging plaque, the laser tends to burn through the artery itself. Now the laser must be "tamed."

There are new drug therapies on the horizon as well. One of the drugs that scientists in Los Angeles are experimenting with works very much like a kitchen drain declogger, eating away plaque in the arteries before blockages occur. So far, the news is encouraging. Several ninety-year-olds who have taken the drug for more than 10 years are still going strong, and the only side effect that any of them has experienced is mild indigestion. (Actually one very famous ninety-year-old who took the drug also fathered a child, but this is probably a coincidence, not a side effect.)

Other treatments for heart disease are being proposed even as you read these words. Naturally, many will fail, but even they may have some value. Today's dreams may save lives tomorrow. I look to a time when we will be so advanced in our knowledge of heart disease that we will be able to prevent it altogether, but even in my most optimistic moments I know that such a time is very far away indeed. Although we have made great progress, in truth we're only beginning to understand why heart disease occurs. We're still a long way from a heart disease-free society.

6

The Heart Patient's Pharmacy

We're all familiar with the cliché: A man has a heart attack, and the next thing you know he's sitting in a wheelchair with a shawl draped around his shoulders and a blanket across his knees. His nurse wakes him every few minutes to give him his medication. Thanks to the miracle of heart surgery and medication, that cliché has gone the way of the horse and buggy. Today's recovering heart patients are not only mobile; if they take care of themselves, they can live very vigorous lives.

One thing hasn't changed, though. Chances are the patient will still have to take some sort of medication. Almost all heart patients will be taking anything from 1 or 2 to 30 or 40 pills a day. Don't regard medication as a sign of weakness or failure; think of it in the same way you think about your healthy diet and your exercise program—as a weapon in your battle against heart disease.

Naturally, your doctor is the expert when it comes to medication; you should always take what's prescribed. But it's a good idea to get to know something about your medicines. Learn what each one does, what the possible side effects are, and how to recognize when they're not doing what they're supposed to be doing. The information in this chapter covers the basics, including a description of the common heart medications, but you should be aware that because every patient is different, every patient's medication will be different. If the information given here differs from what your doctor has told you, ask him or her to clarify the inconsistencies.

BETA BLOCKERS

Perhaps the most commonly prescribed of the heart medications are beta blockers, which block the effect of certain natural heart stimulants on the beta receptors found in the heart and some blood vessels. As a result, the heart is slowed down—your heart rate is lowered by about a third—and your blood pressure is reduced. Beta blockers can play a very important part in cardiac rehabilitation.

Doctors will usually prescribe a beta blocker (to be taken in pill form, two to six times a day) for the treatment of angina, arrhythmia, and hypertension, but equally often they'll prescribe it as a preventive measure. Beta blockers have proved to be very effective; studies show that the recovering heart patient on a beta blocker is one-third less likely to have another heart attack than one who isn't taking a beta blocker. It has also been shown that these drugs dramatically reduce mortality rates for many patients.

If your doctor has prescribed a beta blocker, be sure to take it exactly as you're told, and always ask your doctor's permission before discontinuing beta blocker therapy. One study at the University of California at Davis concluded that for some patients, a withdrawal from medication led to, or worsened, angina or resulted in palpitations and headaches. If it does become necessary to discontinue beta blocker use, your doctor will probably suggest you do so gradually.

CARDIOTONIC GLYCOSIDES

Cardiotonic glycosides, which improve the heart's efficiency, are among the oldest heart drugs still in use. Their discovery dates back to the 1700s, when scientists recognized that medicines derived from the garden plant *digitalis purpurea,* or foxglove, had beneficial effects on the heart when used in subtle dosages.

When it has been damaged by a serious attack, the heart normally speeds up so that blood can be kept flowing throughout the body. However, this doesn't work, since the racing heart does not allow its chambers to fill up with enough new blood between beats. Cardiotonic glycosides, which are taken in pill form once or twice a day, work to reduce the number of times the damaged heart beats, making sure that the chambers fill with a sufficient amount of blood before pumping it to the rest of the body.

There are several types of cardiotonic glycosides now available. Each one is different, in how quickly it takes effect, how long its effects last, and how it is eliminated from the body. In fact, patients may tolerate one cardiotonic glycoside but have problems with another form.

Cardiotonic glycosides should be taken the same time each day. If you forget to take a pill, call your doctor. Don't stop taking cardiotonic glycosides unless you're directed to do so by your doctor. Also, do not take diuretics with cardiotonic glycosides unless your doctor says so. Diuretics can reduce the potassium in your blood, which in turn may increase the toxicity of the cardiotonic glycoside you are taking. Finally, do not take any over-the-counter drugs without consulting your doctor. Many of them, such as cold remedies, nose drops, and laxatives, affect the action of these medications.

ANTIARRHYTHMICS

As you know from chapter 3, arrhythmias are abnormal heart rhythms, which occur when the heart beats in uneven cycles or in an uncoordinated manner. Sometimes arrhythmias are caused by injuries to the heart muscle, or they may occur because of a chemical imbalance, thyroid disease, or an adverse reaction to certain drugs.

Because there are so many different causes for arrhythmias, and because arrhythmias affect different areas of the heart, there are many different antiarrhythmic drugs. This family of drugs works by stabilizing the heart's natural rhythms and controlling irregular heartbeats. Your doctor may want to start you off on a series of antiarrhythmics to see which your body tolerates best. The daily dose may be anything from a pill once a day to one every three hours.

Antiarrhythmic medications must be taken under strict medical supervision, since some may produce severe side effects, such as vomiting, arthritis, muscle twitching, asthma, and blood disorders.

NITRATES

Nitrates are prescribed to relieve the pain of angina, which is the heart's way of telling you it is not getting enough oxygen. If you've ever experienced an angina attack, you know it can be very distressing. Nitrates are vasodilators, meaning they dilate (or widen) blood vessels, thereby allowing more blood to flow toward the heart and quickly replenishing it with badly needed oxygen. The most commonly prescribed form of nitrate is nitroglycerin, and it is available in several forms: tablet, spray, paste, or patch.

Nitroglycerin Tablets

Most people take their nitroglycerin in the form of a tablet placed under the tongue or upper lip or against the cheek and allowed to dissolve. The drug works quickly (within 10 minutes or so) to lessen the heart's workload and to relieve the discomfort of angina.

Nitroglycerin is not habit forming, so don't hesitate to use it whenever you think it is necessary. (It's also not explosive, which is what one of my patients who had seen too many old movies was worried about. He used to carry his pills around in a lead container!) The best time to take nitroglycerin is as soon as the sensation of discomfort starts. To be on the safe side, you may choose to take a tablet just before you engage in an activity that you know is going to cause discomfort.

Nitroglycerin tablets may lose their effectiveness after a relatively short period of time, so it's wise to purchase only a small amount of the drug at a time, and don't keep any nitroglycerin tablets for longer than six months after the date of purchase. The best way to be sure that your medication stays fresh is to keep the tablets in the airtight, moisture-proof dark brown bottle that they came in. After you open the bottle, discard the cotton filler in the bottle; it can interfere with the potency of the drug. Once a week, take out four or five fresh tablets and carry them in another brown glass container in a pocket or in your handbag. At the end of each week, throw out the nitroglycerin tablets you were carrying and take some new ones from your stock.

Don't store nitroglycerin in the inside pocket of your clothes, your bathroom medicine cabinet, the glove compartment of your car, near a fireplace, or in any other hot or humid location. Its effectiveness will be best retained if it's stored at a temperature of about 70°F (21°C). In the summer, consider storing your medication in the refrigerator.

Hospital emergency department staff members often see patients who have suffered an angina attack, taken their nitroglycerin, and become frightened because they obtained no relief. These patients think they're having a heart attack, but all that has happened is that their nitroglycerin has gotten stale.

Always play it safe. You can tell nitroglycerin tablets are fresh if they produce a slight burning sensation after you have placed them in your mouth. If your discomfort continues after you've taken two or three nitroglycerin tablets, immediately contact the paramedics or have someone drive you to the nearest hospital. There is always the possibility that you are really having another heart attack and need immediate emergency care.

Nitroglycerin Spray

If you have been prescribed nitroglycerin in spray form, you will use it in much the same way that others use tablets. One puff of the spray aimed at the roof of your mouth is equivalent to taking one tablet. The spray is faster-acting than tablets, and it has a longer shelf life. However, because it is not possible to control the exact dose with a spray, many doctors are reluctant to prescribe it.

Nitroglycerin Paste

Nitroglycerin paste was very popular in the 1930s, but very few people still use it. It's easy enough to use—it's just applied to the chest and forgotten—but it's messy, and it tends to soil clothing.

Nitroglycerin Patches

Those patients who are prescribed nitroglycerin patches must wear the patch taped to their skin on the upper torso at all times in order for the medication to be properly absorbed. These patches are no bigger than a matchbook and are usually waterproof. They must be changed every 12 hours. However, even if you are wearing the patch, you will need to take a nitroglycerin tablet in case of an angina attack. Medication is absorbed too slowly from the patch to be effective during an angina attack. There's also a chance that your body will develop a tolerance for the patch, which means that the nitroglycerin will no longer be effective in the treatment of an angina attack. If this happens, your doctor will have to discontinue the patches and prescribe nitroglycerin in another form.

Isosorbide Dinitrate

Another nitrate sometimes used in the treatment of angina is isosorbide dinitrate. This drug acts for a much longer period of time than nitroglycerin and is often prescribed when the effect of a nitrate is required around the clock.

DIURETICS

Diuretics, which help rid the body of excess fluids, are often used to treat edema. Edema occurs when the heart's pumping action fails, and blood and fluid collect in the legs and arms. If your doctor prescribes diuretics, you must take the pills regularly and exactly as directed. Do not use the medications only when you're feeling bloated. Ask your physician about taking diuretics before bedtime. Many people experience insomnia with these drugs, because they need to go to the bathroom several times during the night. Be sure to weigh yourself daily to make sure you're not retaining or losing too much fluid. Contact your doctor if you experience an inexplicable weight gain or loss of more than three pounds in a day.

Avoid salt when you are taking diuretics and make sure you get enough potassium, which is lost every time you urinate. Potassium-rich foods include prunes, peaches, dates, raisins, potatoes, and bananas. If you lose a lot of potassium—some signs are lethargy and muscle cramps—your doctor may prescribe potassium chloride to replace it. Potassium chloride is slightly unpleasant in taste, but it's necessary for recovery.

ANTICOAGULANTS

When your blood clots, it blocks blood circulation, which may in turn cause a heart attack, pulmonary embolism, even a stroke. Anticoagulants "thin" the blood in order to prevent clots. For obvious reasons, you have to be very careful when you take these drugs. Since your blood is not clotting as it would under normal conditions, you must avoid anything that might cause accidental bleeding. I tell my patients to shave with an electric razor instead of a blade, use a soft toothbrush, and always wear shoes. I recommend a plastic mat in the bathtub to help you avoid slipping.

If you notice any unusual bleeding or bruising, notify your doctor at once. Call too if you see blood in your urine or stool, if you experience nosebleeds, or if you have a heavier than normal menstrual flow. You should undergo frequent blood samples to make sure your anticoagulant dosage is correct.

Anticoagulants and many prescription and nonprescription drugs don't mix. Be sure to check every medication you take with your doctor. Careless experimentation could threaten your life.

Effects of Aspirin

In recent years, aspirin has been found to inhibit the blood's clotting action. As a result, many doctors, myself among them, are now prescribing an aspirin a day as an anticoagulant agent for patients who have had a heart attack and are at risk of experiencing another one. However, you must not take aspirin or an ibuprofen product, such as Advil or Nuprin, if you are on another anticoagulant prescribed by your doctor. Since aspirin has its own anticlotting abilities, the combination of it and another anticoagulant may interfere with your body's ability to stop accidental bleeding.

CALCIUM CHANNEL BLOCKERS

Calcium channel blockers are similar to nitrates, and like nitrates, they are prescribed to treat angina. (One type, verapamil, is sometimes used to treat arrhythmias.) Although it is not known exactly why these drugs work, we do know that they relieve the pain of angina by inhibiting the passage of calcium ions across cell membranes. We also know that each calcium channel blocker works a little differently, so you may have to try a few before you find one that works well for you.

Some patients may be prescribed both a calcium channel blocker and a beta blocker or a calcium channel blocker and a nitrate to relieve angina. The dose is usually two pills a day.

All calcium channel blockers should be used with extreme caution, especially if you have low blood pressure or are taking low blood pressure medication. It is a good idea to have your blood pressure routinely monitored while on these medications.

OTHER MEDICATIONS

Anxiety, muscle cramping, and constipation may be related to heart disease and its treatment. Should you experience these or other problems, your doctor may prescribe other drugs, such as stool softeners and muscle relaxants, along with those normally recommended for treating disease. Again, follow your doctor's orders at all times. Do not try to cure your problems with over-the-counter drugs before checking with a physician. Mixing heart drugs even with what seems like harmless store-bought remedies could be very dangerous.

FOUR IMPORTANT PIECES OF ADVICE

1. **Make sure that your prescriptions are up to date.** For example, say you had a touch of heart failure. You were considerably overweight, and your doctor recommended a diuretic. Then you went into a cardiac rehabilitation program, tuned up your body, and lost quite a bit of weight. Chances are you no longer need the diuretic, but you still have a prescription for it. Frankly, your doctor may have forgotten that he or she prescribed it. If you suspect that you no longer need to take a given medication, ask your doctor about it. In fact, every six months you should have a "medication update." If your doctor doesn't initiate a discussion you should do so.
2. **Never give your medication to another person or take someone else's prescription.** If your doctor stops prescribing a particular medicine, flush it down the toilet so it will not be used by anyone else or fall into the hands of curious children. Thousands of children die every year because adults leave their medications lying around. Although heart medications can save your life, they are extremely dangerous if used improperly or by the wrong person.
3. **Remember that medications can lose their effectiveness.** If you have discontinued the use of a

medication and then your doctor starts it up again, always buy a new bottle, especially if the medicine is nitroglycerin.

4. **Carry an identification card that specifies which drugs you are taking.** (Medic Alert makes one). This will help you in an emergency or if you lose your medication while traveling and need to refill your prescription.

THE FUTURE OF MEDICATION

There is no question in my mind that as far as drug therapy for heart disease is concerned, there is good news coming in the years ahead. Our knowledge is increasing practically every day. In the last several years, more medications were introduced for the treatment of heart disease than ever before. What's more, researchers are continuing to make discoveries about the medications already available to the public. For instance, the use of aspirin as a heart medication was discovered only recently, and new research reveals that beta blockers and calcium channel blockers may have more than one application in heart disease treatment. Calcium channel blockers seem to be effective in helping the damaged heart heal after a heart attack; beta blockers could be critical for preventing another heart attack and sudden death.

What does all this tell you, the patient? It tells you to keep a positive attitude about what lies ahead. It is quite possible that you could benefit from much of the drug research being conducted right now.

CHART OF HEART MEDICATIONS

The chart on the following pages outlines the purpose, usage instructions, and side effects of most common heart medications. Use it for quick reference, but if you need further information, be sure to contact your doctor.

HEART MEDICATIONS

Medication	Instructions	Purpose of Medication	Side Effects	Side Effects to Report to Doctor
Cardiotonic Glycosides				
Digitalis		Increases the heart's ability to pump more effectively; controls arrhythmias		Nausea and vomiting; new heart palpitations
Digoxin (Lanoxin)				
Diuretics				
Furosemide (Lasix)	If on one dose a day, take in the morning	Helps rid the body of extra fluid		Weakness; dizziness; leg cramps; loss of appetite
Dyazide				
Hydrochlorthiazide (Hydrodiuril)				
Potassium				
KCL (potassium chloride)	Bitter tasting—may mix with juice	Replaces potassium the body loses when taking a diuretic (potassium is necessary for normal heart function)	May cause stomach upset if not mixed with juice	Weakness; dizziness; leg cramps; loss of appetite; diarrhea

Nitrates				
NTG (nitroglycerin) Isosorbide dinitrate (Sorbitrate, Isordil sublingual, oral, chewable)	Place under the tongue; let it dissolve; may be repeated every 5 min. if chest pain is not relieved; do not drink water with this pill	To relieve chest pain (heaviness or tightness in the chest)	Headache, temporary warm flushed feeling or dizziness; temporary weak feeling; faster pulse	If chest pain is not relieved after 2–3 tablets (1 every 5 min.), call doctor and paramedics; or go to emergency dept.
	Note: May be taken prior to activity you feel may cause chest pain Keep nitroglycerin in original bottle for maximum freshness. Use new bottle every 3–6 months as directed.			
Antiarrhythmics				
Disopyramide (Norpace)		Helps the heart beat more regularly	Blurred vision; urinary hesitancy; nausea	Urinary retention; fainting; dizziness
Quinidine	Take with milk or meals to avoid stomach (gastric) irritation			Nausea; loss of appetite; dizziness; skin rash; tinnitus

HEART MEDICATIONS (CONTINUED)

Medication	Instructions	Purpose of Medication	Side Effects	Side Effects to Report to Doctor
Antiarrhythmics (continued)				
Meiletine (Meitil) Procainamide (Pronestyl) Tocainide (Tonocard) Flecainide (Tambocor)			Light-headedness	Muscular aches or pain; dizziness; skin rash; tremors or blurred vision; gastrointestinal distress; palpitations blood problems
Beta Blockers				
Propranolol (Inderal) Timolol (Blocadre) Metoprolol (Lopressor) Nadolol (Corgard) Atenolol (Tenormin)	Do not discontinue medication without first consulting physician	Decreases blood pressure; helps to keep the heart rhythm regular; helps to relieve chest pain; may help prevent further heart attacks		Dizziness; light-headedness; shortness of breath; ankle swelling; wheezing; weakness

Anticoagulants				
Sulfinpyrazone (Anturane)	Take with milk to avoid stomach (gastric) irritation	Thought to decrease clotting in vessels by effect on platelets; may help prevent further heart attacks	Nausea; gastrointestinal upset	Rash; bleeding
Dipyridamole (Persantine)				
Aspirin	Try an enteric coated product that dissolves slowly in the gastrointestinal tract			
Wafarin sodium (Coumadin)	Take as directed by physician; have regular blood tests; avoid aspirin; consult with physician or pharmacist before taking over-the-counter drugs	Prolongs clotting of blood		Bleeding; bruising; blood in urine; black or bloody stools; nose bleeding

HEART MEDICATIONS (CONTINUED)

Medication	Instructions	Purpose of Medication	Side Effects	Side Effects to Report to Doctor
Calcium Channel Blockers				
Verapamil (Isoptin, Calan) Nifedipine (Procardia) Diltiazem (Cardizem)	May interact with digoxin or blood pressure medicines	Decreases the severity and frequency of angina; reduces coronary spasm	Constipation; headache; heartburn; flushing	Dizziness; giddiness; fainting
Other Medications				
Pentoifylline (Trental)	Take after meals for intermittent clodication	Improves leg cramps (but takes several weeks to work)	Gastrointestinal upset	Extreme gastrointestinal upset; chest pain; dizziness; headache
Diazepam (Valium)	Do not take with alcohol	To relax muscles and relieve tension or anxiety	Sleepiness; fatigue; occasionally blurred vision when reading	
Stool softener (e.g., D.S.S., Colace)	Daily or as needed; avoid taking with mineral oil	Prevents straining at bowel movements		Diarrhea

Source: Compiled by author.

7

Outpatient Cardiac Rehabilitation Programs

Let me tell you my favorite medical story. It happened some years ago, when a middle-aged man who had been ill for some time went to see his doctor. After giving the patient a thorough examination, the doctor had no choice but to tell the man the bad news: He had inoperable cancer. As a matter of fact, his body was riddled with cancer; as far as the doctor could determine, the patient had less than a month to live. Naturally the man got a second opinion, and then a third, but everyone said the same thing. The cancer was untreatable. Death was imminent. He was given a supply of painkillers and sent home.

About two years later the doctor got a call from his patient. The man said he was sorry to bother the doctor, but he wanted to know if there was anything he should be doing about his health. He felt fine, he said, but he was confused. Was it okay for him to go back to work? What about traveling? After all, he hadn't expected to be alive this long.

Naturally the doctor was stunned, and he asked the man to come in that very day for an examination. By the time the patient got to the doctor's office, a crowd of doctors had gathered. When they examined the man, they discovered that the cancer had completely disappeared. There was nothing wrong with the man. No one had any idea what had happened.

I think that the reason I like this story so much—and it's well documented, by the way—is because it's the best example I know of the body's remarkable healing abilities. In some ways it's the ultimate rehabilitation story.

As the director of a cardiac rehabilitation center I have collected lots of good recovery stories. Most of them aren't quite so dramatic, but they're all satisfying. As you can imagine, I am all in favor of formal cardiac rehabilitation programs; I think that everyone who has had a heart attack should go through some sort of cardiac rehabilitation. While it is certainly possible to recover your health without a formal, supervised program, there is no question in my mind that it brings about better, faster results.

WHAT THEY DO

It's quite simple: Outpatient cardiac rehabilitation programs help heart attack patients achieve complete recovery and assist them in forming new, healthy life-styles. They also do something that is not so simple: They lift the spirit and inspire a sense of camaraderie. The people participating in cardiac rehabilitation programs offer one another friendship, support, and encouragement during a difficult time.

Most programs involve three exercise sessions per week, during which you strengthen your heart through a gradually accelerating program of activity. In addition to assisting with your physical recovery, the programs meet other needs, such as psychological counseling, physical therapy, dietary guidance, and occupational therapy. Usually these services are available through the program at an additional, but minimal, cost.

HOW TO CHOOSE A PROGRAM

There's more than one way to rehabilitate a heart. Cardiac rehabilitation centers range from places that allow people to run unmonitored around a track with a defibrillator to live-in programs in which the patient's every move is monitored. Some are affiliated with a hospital; others are independent.

Your hospital may have a program of its own. If you had some inpatient cardiac rehabilitation during your hospital stay, that program may require you to return to the hospital as often as three times a week during your convalescent phase. If there is no formal program associated with your hospital, you'll have to find one on your own. You won't have to look far for advice, though. Doctors, nurses, social workers, and other hospital personnel will be willing and able to point you in the right direction.

I can't choose a specific program for you. What I can do is tell you what I think constitutes a good program:

- **Medical supervision.** Your medical progress will be monitored by your own doctor during cardiac rehabilitation, but the medical director of the center should be aware of every aspect of your condition. The center should have copies of the results of all of the tests you have been given, including stress tests, cardiac catheterization, and tests for diabetes, cholesterol, and triglyceride levels. The center should have the facilities to administer a mini–stress test and a full stress test whenever your doctor believes they are called for.

- **Education.** There should be a structured environment in which you can learn about the care and feeding of your heart.
- **Psychological counseling.** A psychiatrist, a psychologist, or a psychotherapist should be available to talk to you about any problems you are encountering during recovery. These same professionals will have advice on how you can avoid and control stress.
- **Physical therapy.** One of the most important aspects of cardiac rehabilitation is a structured, sensible exercise program. There should be someone on staff to advise you and monitor your progress.
- **Nutritional counseling.** Obesity is an important risk factor in heart disease, so weight control is critical in any cardiac rehabilitation program. You may have been advised to follow a special low-salt, low-fat, or low-cholesterol diet. There should be a registered dietitian on staff to give you advice and check on your progress.
- **Occupational therapy.** On rare occasions you may have to relearn some basic skills to accommodate a temporary weakness. An occupational therapist should be there to help you.
- **Vocational guidance.** Many people recovering from a heart attack seriously consider changing jobs. There should be an expert on call with whom you can discuss the physical and emotional ramifications of a job change.
- **Family therapy.** You and your loved ones are in this thing together, and there will be times when you'll want

to talk with a professional about any problems the family is having. A good cardiac rehabilitation program will have facilities for family therapy.

WHEN, HOW LONG, AND HOW MUCH?

As far as I'm concerned, cardiac rehabilitation starts the moment you realize that you've been through a heart attack and you're not going to die. Most formal programs begin right after a patient leaves the hospital and starts the convalescence period and may last from anywhere between three and six months. Be sure to follow the plan exactly as it is prescribed for you. If you are meant to go in three times a week for five months, stick to your schedule.

PERSONNEL

As I've already said, all cardiac rehabilitation centers are different, but the typical center will have the following professionals in addition to the front-office staff: a medical director; registered (usually cardiac) nurses; a registered dietitian; a social worker; a psychiatrist or psychologist; a physical therapist; and an occupational therapist.

SOME GOOD NEWS

I began this chapter with one of my favorite stories. I will end it with the result of a study conducted a few years ago by our heart research team.

One hundred heart attack victims were closely monitored from the moment they entered the hospital until exactly a year later. We discovered that a patient's physical condition—blood pressure, stress test results, level of physical activity, and so forth—twelve months after a heart attack has nothing whatever to do with the severity of the heart attack or how sick the patient had been before it happened. What it does have to do with is what has been done for the patient's health since the attack.

If that's not an argument for cardiac rehabilitation, I don't know what is.

8

Leaving the Hospital

Finally, you're ready to go home! No more hospital gowns, no more hospital food, no more longing for your own bed. It's time for all the comforts of home, not to mention a little privacy.

There are lots of reasons to be happy just now, the most important of which is that you've made it past a very crucial part of your recovery. You no longer need constant care. Now you can start recuperating on your own, or almost on your own. You'll need a little help from your family or perhaps a nurse. All things considered, though, things are really looking up.

But before you pack your belongings and get ready for the wheelchair ride out the front door of the hospital, you have some important business to attend to. In fact, here's a list of things to do before you take your leave.

1. **Make an appointment.** Make your next doctor's appointment before you leave the hospital. Ask for the name of someone you might call for assistance just in case your doctor is off duty. Most doctors have other doctors covering for them during weekends and vacations. For your own peace of mind, get their names.

2. **Know your medication.** Before you leave, make sure that you have all the medication you will need for the next few weeks and that you know what each medicine is for, how it should be taken, what the possible side effects are, and what you should do if they occur. On a card small enough to fit in your wallet, write your doctor's name and telephone number on one side and a list of the medications you are taking (complete with dosage instructions) on the back. (For more information about medications see chapter 6.)
3. **Ask about food restrictions.** If you are supposed to be on a special diet, make sure you know all the details. If the diet sounds confusing or difficult to follow, ask to see the dietitian before you leave the hospital. Substitutions can often be made.
4. **Think about a cardiac rehabilitation program.** If you think that you'll be joining a cardiac rehabilitation program any time during your recovery period, now is the time to make arrangements. You should be starting the program as soon as you get home. The program you choose may be affiliated with the hospital you're in, another hospital, or a doctor's practice closer to home. Regardless of which one you pick, make an appointment to visit the hospital and talk to the staff as soon as possible. You will want to be sure that the arrangements there are convenient and well suited to your tastes and needs. (See chapter 7 for more about cardiac rehabilitation programs.)
5. **Look into home nursing assistance.** Some local government or community authorities have services that may entitle you to free nursing assistance at home if you are incapacitated. If you would like this type of service, ask the hospital social worker about it before leaving the hospital. Other professionals, such as physical therapists, occupational therapists, pharmacists, psychiatrists, and psychologists, usually are available through these services. If you would like a follow-up outpatient appointment with any one of them, make arrangements before you check out.

6. **Ask questions.** This is a good time to ask your doctor for practical advice on how you should handle daily activities, such as driving, traveling, walking, managing stairs, engaging in sex, and doing housework. Make sure to write down questions when you think of them so that you will not forget them.
7. **Know your risk factors.** Risk factors, which include obesity, high blood pressure, stress, diabetes, and smoking, affect your chances of having another heart attack. Before you go home, ask your doctor's opinion about which of these conditions applies to your situation and what you should do about them. (See chapter 10 for a complete discussion of risk factors.)
8. **Know how to use nitroglycerin.** If your doctor has prescribed nitroglycerin, be sure you know how to use it properly. Oral nitroglycerin may deteriorate rapidly, so you should find out how to make sure you'll always have a fresh supply.
9. **For pacemaker wearers.** If you had a permanent pacemaker implanted during your stay, you should add the type of pacemaker and its year of manufacture to the medication card you have in your wallet. I advise many of my patients to wear an identification bracelet, and your doctor may think that's the best course for you. Ask about it before you leave the hospital.

9

The Convalescent Phase

When a woman goes home after having a baby, she often experiences what obstetricians call the "third-day blues." The birth of her child was a great high. Flowers arrived, relatives called, and her husband was constantly by her side. Then she goes home. Three days later, her husband goes back to work, the flowers have wilted, and the dirty diapers have started to mount up. It's not unusual for the new mother to sit down and have a good cry.

The heart patient often has the same kinds of feelings when he or she leaves the hospital and goes home. I conducted a study among my patients and found that approximately 35 out of every 100 heart attack patients were depressed when they went home. In about 9 of these 35 cases, the depression required special medication or counseling. I also concluded that about one-fourth of all heart attack patients experience some degree of anxiety.

It's easy to understand why the heart patient has mixed

emotions as the convalescent phase begins. On the one hand, the patient is incredibly happy to be alive and out of the hospital; on the other, now that all the excitement is over, the patient may be realizing for the first time that he or she is really sick. Sometimes patients feel depressed because even though they don't feel any discomfort, their activities are still curtailed.

WHAT IS HAPPENING PHYSICALLY

One of the best ways to snap out of a temporary feeling of letdown is to understand what is happening to you physically during the convalescent phase. Basically, the heart muscle is forming a total and complete scar, a process that takes approximately six weeks. The body essentially heals itself, provided it is not injured any further.

And that's really what convalescence is all about—making sure that the body is allowed to heal itself without sustaining any further injury. During this healing period you will gradually increase your activities, and the damaged area of your heart will become stronger and better able to endure increased activity. For obvious reasons, anything that might impede the formation of the scar tissue must be avoided during this time. Some patients are entirely healed in 6 weeks, but others take as long as 12 weeks. Only your doctor can judge how well you're progressing.

Many patients become concerned that the damaged area of the heart will still be "soft" or "mushy" even after convalescence is finished. It won't. At the end of your convalescence, the affected area will be as strong as the unaffected areas of your heart. Only on rare occasions will its contour differ from the rest of the heart muscle.

• • •

GAME PLAN FOR CONVALESCENCE

Some patients regard the convalescent period as a welcome opportunity to rest, catch up on their reading, watch television, paint, or pursue other hobbies. Others look upon it as a prisoner might regard a cell. If you were a very active person before your heart attack, relaxing may be quite a foreign activity. Chances are you didn't even consider taking an occasional breather before your heart attack. Perhaps the best way for you to adjust to such an extreme change in activity, then, is to take greater interest in things you never had the time to do before.

Try reading the whole newspaper from beginning to end, take up gourmet cooking, work in the darkroom, start a stamp collection. Anything that keeps your interest and is not physically demanding will do the trick. Some people take this time to review their plans for retirement, treating this recovery period as a sort of practice run for the years when they'll be completely free to pursue interests they did not have time for during their working lives. Others who have hopes of setting up a small shop or business upon retirement can use the recovery period for mapping out a plan.

As you watch other family members going to work, you may feel guilty about not working. This is normal. Don't call the office five times a day just to check up on things. It's fine to stay in touch with your job but don't be like one workaholic patient I had. When I visited him in his hospital room ten days after he had been admitted for a heart attack, he was dictating memos to not one but two secretaries. Perhaps it will help you to think of this time as a vacation. In fact, you might use the time to make plans for a real vacation when you are strong enough.

Like most things in life, convalescence is what you make of it. Here are a few hints for making sure yours runs smoothly:

- Take things slowly. Do not think you must immediately return to your normal life-style.

- Take a long, hard look at the way you've been living your life. Now is the time to give up unhealthy habits and build positive, healthy ones.

- Consider your convalescence as a time devoted to building confidence in yourself. Although it may seem as if you are progressing very slowly at first, do not despair. Each week will produce more and more visible change.

- Educate yourself. The more you know about how you can help yourself, the more progress you will make during this important convalescent stage. Read and ask questions.

- Remember that it is extremely important to listen to your doctor right now. Every individual's condition is unique, and your own physician may provide you with some special guidance that is particularly important for your case. Well-meaning friends or relatives will offer advice, but don't act on it until you've spoken to your doctor. Once a patient told me that a nurse he was dating said it was okay for him to start jogging as soon as he felt up to it. Of course, I couldn't show him how angry I was, since he was flat on his back in the cardiac care unit.

- Join (or even start) a small support group of people who are in a situation similar to yours. Your doctor will be able to introduce you to other convalescing heart patients.

- Above all, remember that your goal is complete recovery, with limited changes in your life-style. Focusing on this goal will remind you why you are taking life a bit more slowly. Convalescence may be frustrating, but eventually it will pay off.

Now, let's discuss the specifics of your convalescent program for the next four to six weeks.

GROUND RULES FOR CONVALESCENCE

In general, there are certain activities you should definitely avoid during your convalescent period, such as lifting, pulling, or pushing anything heavy. Your doctor will usually permit you to lift parcels of about 10 pounds or less during the first two weeks. During the third and fourth weeks, you can probably progress to 20 pounds. By the end of the convalescent phase, you'll probably be beyond 30 pounds.

Be sure to ask your doctor about sex. Most patients are permitted to resume sexual activity after a short time of convalescence, but each case is different. (See chapter 11 for more details on sex and the heart patient.)

In fact, you should discuss every aspect of your convalescent program with your doctor, and if you are attending an outpatient cardiac rehabilitation program, talk to the staff there too. Their advice will reinforce the information offered in this book as well as the advice given you by your doctor. Once you have spoken to your doctor and cardiac rehabilitation team, try incorporating these general points into the program they recommend:

1. Lying around all day in your pajamas is bad for your morale. It will only make you feel like an invalid, which you are not. Every day you should get out of bed, get dressed, shave, fix your hair, put on makeup, and so forth.
2. The first couple of days at home should be about as active as your last day at the hospital. After that you should increase your activity level gradually. Take a half hour to a full hour's rest twice a day during your first two

weeks at home. During the next two weeks, rest once a day or any time you get tired. Space out your activities appropriately, alternating between rest and moving around.

3. Identify the risk factors in your life and create a plan for eliminating them. Stop smoking. Follow your diet. Do not add salt to your food unless your doctor or dietitian permits it. Do your exercises and take a walk every day, but be sure to wait for at least an hour after eating before exercising.
4. Beware of extremes in temperature. Showers are preferable to baths, and they should be warm, not very hot or very cold. Do not shower immediately after exercise. If you do take a bath, don't spend a long time in the tub, and again, use warm water. Be very careful the first few times you bathe after your heart attack; many people get dizzy when stepping out of the tub. Check with your doctor before traveling to a very hot or humid place, a very cold place, or before using a sauna, whirlpool, or steambath.
5. Take your medicine exactly as your doctor ordered. Refill your prescriptions before you run out of medicine. If you don't have the prescription order, contact your doctor.
6. Keep your medical appointments. If possible, have someone accompany you on the first few visits.
7. Weigh yourself daily. If your weight shoots up three or more pounds in one day and doesn't come down the next, call your doctor.
8. Take special precautions with stairs. Plan your day so that you don't have to climb stairs unnecessarily. If your bedroom is upstairs, check with your doctor about sleeping downstairs. If you are told to try managing the stairs, climb them only once or twice a day. During the first week of stair-climbing, take only a few steps at a time, stopping to rest for a few seconds before continuing. Later you can go up and down slowly without stopping.

9. Stop what you are doing if you feel pain in your chest, shoulder, arm, neck, or jaws; dizziness; or shortness of breath. Take your nitroglycerin (if your doctor prescribed it for you) and rest for several minutes. When the discomfort goes away, continue what you were doing at a slower rate. If it does not go away after 15 minutes of rest and/or two nitroglycerin tablets, have someone drive you to the nearest hospital emergency department or call the paramedics.
10. Don't drive a car without your doctor's permission. During the first two weeks after your heart attack, try to travel only a short distance in the car with someone else driving. Later, you may drive short distances only if someone is in the passenger seat next to you. Avoid freeway driving as much as possible. Check with your doctor before taking a long trip in a car. If you have to travel a long distance, stop every hour or two and walk around. This will prevent blood clots from forming in your legs.
11. Notify your doctor if you experience *any* of the following: chest or arm discomfort at short, frequent intervals lasting for about 30 seconds; increased shortness of breath; unusual fatigue; swollen feet or ankles; fainting spells; very slow or rapid heart rate; unusual palpitations.

BODY MECHANICS

Knowing basic body mechanics will help you conserve energy and prevent injury during the convalescent phase. Remember, anything that makes your heart work too hard will hinder the critical healing process, and it may even bring on angina or heart palpitations. It may be difficult to change the way you go about your simple daily activities—after all, you're not used to thinking about them—but every little change can help.

1. **Getting out of bed.** Before you try to sit up, turn on your side and lower your legs off the bed as you use your arms

to push yourself into a sitting position. Keep your spine very straight. This is called "getting up like a chair." When you go back to bed, simply reverse the motion.

2. **Getting out of a chair.** Move toward the edge of the chair, position your feet directly under you, and push up with your legs, keeping your back very straight.
3. **Sitting.** Always sit erect in a chair with both feet flat on the floor, knee-level with your hips. It may be wise to avoid your favorite overstuffed chair for a few weeks. Straight-backed chairs may be less comfortable, but at the moment they're better for you.
4. **Bending.** When you pick something up off the floor, never bend from the waist. Bend your knees and go into a squat, keeping your back as straight as possible.
5. **Carrying.** You may not be permitted to carry anything for a while. When your doctor does allow it, always carry things in both hands and close to your body.
6. **Reaching.** If you must reach (avoid it whenever possible), don't overreach. You may become dizzy if you put your arms over your head. Make sure you are as close to the object as you can get before you reach for it; for instance, stand on a stool when you take dishes out of the kitchen cupboard. Remember that arm activity creates more work for the heart than leg activity.
7. **Driving.** If and when your doctor permits you to drive, adjust the seat so that it's close to the steering wheel. Your knees should be at least as high as your hips. If your back bothers you, change your position so that your knees are even higher.

ENERGY CONSERVATION

Like a knowledge of body dynamics, a familiarity with how your body uses energy can be very useful during the convalescent phase. On the one hand, you need to expend some energy—you'll be getting some exercise every day—but on the other, the wrong kind of energy expenditure can overwork the heart. These tips on energy conservation will be helpful in your daily activities.

1. **Analyze each activity before you start.** Ask yourself some basic questions: What materials do I need? Are they close at hand or will I have to make several trips to retrieve them? How much cleanup is required? Can I handle it? Always look for shortcuts. Eliminate unnecessary steps and simplify others.
2. **Reorganize your life.** Have someone rearrange your cupboards, dresser drawers, and medicine cabinet so that you can eliminate unnecessary reaching, stooping, or prolonged standing. Store related materials (for example, decaffeinated coffee, sweeteners, cups, spoons, and the coffee brewer) together.
3. **Never rush.** Allow yourself sufficient time to complete a given task and rest afterward.
4. **Rethink your regular routine.** Even if you've been following the same schedule every day for years, you'll do well to make some changes. For instance, sit down while toweling off after a shower, shaving, applying makeup, or drying your hair. This may take some getting used to, but it's worth the effort.

HOUSEHOLD ACTIVITIES

It may be difficult to accept at first, but during convalescence there's no such thing as an activity you can perform without thinking. Even the simplest household chores may present a challenge. The doctor will probably allow light housework, but it's important that you do it very slowly during the first two weeks—no bed making, washing and hanging clothes, or floor scrubbing, please. Desk work is also likely to be allowed. Every chore must be approved by your doctor. Of course, there is a right way and a wrong way to complete a task. Keep the following points in mind as you work around the house.

1. **Save steps.** When you are allowed to start cleaning, finish one room before going on to the next. Make your bed one side at a time. Don't do any unnecessary tasks; you can wash dishes, but don't dry them.
2. **Sit down while washing dishes, ironing, or preparing meals.** Sit on the rim of the bathtub when you clean it and use a long-handled brush.
3. **Don't wash windows, dust in high places, or hang clothes on the line.** Working with your arms above your shoulder makes your heart work harder.
4. **Don't move furniture or lift heavy steel pots and pans.** If you must handle cast iron skillets, slide them. When serving, transfer the food to a serving dish or onto separate plates. Do not try to lift the heavy pot. When you are transferring clothes from the washer to the dryer, lift only one or two articles at a time. Use a dolly to carry out the garbage.
5. **Do not pick up young children during the first few weeks of your convalescence unless absolutely necessary.** This can be very difficult (who can resist a baby, especially one who is crying?), so I suggest to my patients that they hire a babysitter to help out.
6. **Be careful when you're working in the garden.** Don't stoop over to pull weeds; squat or, even better, sit on the ground. When you rake leaves, be sure not to overreach. Mowing the lawn (with either a hand or an electric mower) usually is not allowed during the convalescent stage, but if your doctor says it's all right, again, don't overreach.

SOCIAL ACTIVITIES

Most doctors will want you to start socializing during convalescence, but they'll probably warn you not to do too much too soon. During the first week you'll be encouraged to relax with your immediate family and perhaps talk on the phone for short periods of time. (Long or argumentative phone calls may cause stress.) During the second week you'll probably be allowed to have a few visitors over but only for a short while—no late nights or wild parties. By the third week you'll start going out to dinner. You may be permitted to attend religious services or go to a movie, concert, or play.

By the fourth week things will be getting almost back to normal. You may start having small parties in your home. In the fifth week you'll be permitted to attend club meetings, small picnics, and school activities provided you are not too heavily involved in the activities. It's all right to go to a PTA meeting; it's not all right to run for PTA president.

EXERCISE

During the convalescent phase you will probably be taking short daily walks, with your doctor's approval, of course. I suggest to my patients that they supplement their walk with a few regular exercise routines. The following exercises are simple, and they're designed to prepare you for the more strenuous activities you'll be handling in later phases of your recovery.

Warm-up and Cool-down Exercises

If your doctor gives you permission, do the following routines three times a day: before you go walking (these are your warm-up exercises); immediately after you finish walking (now they're your cool-down exercises); and about 12 hours before you think you'll take your next walk. Carry a copy of these exercises with you until you have committed them to memory.

1. In a standing position, lift yourself up and down on your toes. Repeat 10 times.

2. In a standing position, with your hands on your hips, twist your upper body gently to the left and then to the right. Repeat 10 times.
3. In a standing position, with your hands at your sides and your back straight, bend to the left and then to the right. Repeat 10 times.
4. Bring one leg out to the front, to the side, to the back, and back to the ground. Repeat with other leg. Do each leg 10 more times.
5. March in place for 20 beats.
6. With your feet flat on the floor and your back straight, bend your knees slightly and then straighten up. Repeat 10 times.
7. Bend at the waist and touch your left knee with your right hand. Then touch your right knee with your left hand. Repeat 10 times.

Walking

No matter how great you begin to feel during convalescence, you won't be doing any running, jogging, or swimming for a while. You won't be playing tennis or golf, and you won't be going dancing. The bowling team will have to make it to the championship without you. If all goes well, you'll do all those things and more eventually, but they will have to be reintroduced into your life gradually, after you have finished your convalescent phase.

Yes, you will be exercising during convalescence, but the major physical exertion you'll get is from walking. Now don't confuse this kind of walking with the walking you've been hearing so much about lately; fitness walking (it's also called race walking or aerobic walking) is something else entirely, designed to give you a vigorous aerobic workout. The kind of walking you'll be doing now will be done carefully and slowly, increasing the distance you walk only as your doctor orders.

No matter what sort of exercise you do, don't push too hard. Avoid exercising when you're tired or when you have a bad cold or other illness. Avoid isometric (muscle-building) exercises; they make the body tense up, increasing blood pressure and making the heart work faster. Isometrics include heavy lifting, pulling, push-ups, straining to open a window or jar lid, and straining to have a bowel movement. Never hold your breath during exercise.

Most patients start with a 10-minute daily walk for the first week and then increase the time by 5 minutes for each of the following four to six weeks. Therefore, you should be walking about 30 minutes a day at the end of the convalescent phase. Remember, at this time the whole idea of walking is not to build body strength; that comes later during the conditioning phase (chapter 14). For now, it's easy does it. Here are some other tips about walking:

1. **Take it slow.** Do your warm-up exercises before you start. Then start walking at a slow pace. Increase your speed slightly, after a few minutes. Just before the end of your walk, slow the pace down again. After your walk do your cool-down exercises immediately.
2. **Avoid exercising in extreme temperatures.** The temperature outside should be at least 55°F (13°C) and no more than 80°F (27°C). In the winter, walk in the late morning or early afternoon; in the summer, go out in the early morning or evening. If the weather outside is especially bad, consider walking in an enclosed shopping mall, supermarket, or hotel-motel complex where there is plenty of heat or air conditioning.
3. **Don't walk after eating.** You should not walk or do other exercises for at least one hour after eating.
4. **Walk on level ground.** Steps and hills make your heart work harder and beat faster.
5. **Avoid sudden bursts of activity.** Don't be tempted to

run across the street to beat a traffic light, for instance. Walk at a comfortable, rhythmic pace.

6. **Always wear loose, comfortable clothing and shoes that fit properly.** I've seen some of my patients get carried away with their equipment, buying a closetful of warm-up suits and walking shoes. There is nothing wrong with going on a shopping spree if it makes you happy, but there's also nothing wrong with wearing your old clothes and sneakers. You don't have to dress like an Olympic athlete to benefit from your walking program!
7. **If you experience any chest discomfort or shortness of breath, stop and sit down on a step or curb.** Place nitroglycerin under your tongue (if your doctor has prescribed it for you). Wait until you feel better before starting to walk again. If this is an uncommon occurrence, call your doctor. If the pain does not go away after 15 minutes or 2 nitroglycerin tablets, have someone take you to the nearest emergency department or call the paramedics immediately.

10

Risk Factors

It wasn't all that long ago that people thought jogging was just for health nuts. Smoking was considered highly sophisticated. And for a perfect meal, nothing seemed to fit the bill like a big juicy steak with all the trimmings. To put it mildly, a lot has changed since then.

We now know that smoking, inactivity, and eating high-fat high-cholesterol foods are unhealthy habits. More to the point, there is strong evidence that these unhealthy habits increase your chances of developing serious heart problems. A few years ago the American Heart Association made it official by compiling a list of these *risk factors,* those activities or traits that make some people more *coronary-prone* than others.

Granted, there are people who have experienced heart attacks even though they were free of risk factors. And conversely, some people with all the indications of being coronary-prone remain perfectly healthy. This is because the human body is a complex mechanism, and try as they might, physicians cannot predict precisely all that triggers its breakdowns. But there are some things physicians do know: that if you don't work to reduce the risk factors in your life, you are taking a serious gamble; and that accumulating more risk factors is like *multiplying,* not adding to, your susceptibility.

Your first step in reducing risk factors is identifying those that apply to your life-style. Read through the following sections and consider those on which you need to work. Then discuss your thoughts with your doctor. He or she will undoubtedly have some helpful suggestions.

Risk factors fall into two general categories, those you can't control and those you can control.

UNCONTROLLABLES

I'd like to be able to tell you that your health is completely in your own hands, but that's not entirely true. Studies have shown that some risk factors are entirely out of a patient's control. However, it's important to be aware that these factors could be working against you. Discuss with your doctor the extent to which they may influence your recovery.

Age

Atherosclerosis can begin in even young children, but the disease rarely becomes apparent until the later years. Therefore, the older you get, the more likely you are to experience the effects of atherosclerosis.

Gender

Women who are still menstruating have a much smaller chance of developing coronary artery disease than men of similar age. This finding may be related to the female sex hormones, which seem to protect the body from developing artherosclerosis. However, postmenopausal women catch up with men; they have just as great a chance of developing heart disease as men in the same age group.

Heredity

I think people worry too much about their relatives. It's true that there is some evidence to suggest that heart attacks run in families, but as far as I'm concerned, the facts are misleading. Remember, nearly 2 million Americans have heart attacks each year, so there's a good chance that just about everyone has at least one relative with heart disease.

You should be concerned only if any of your immediate relatives experienced heart attacks in their twenties or thirties. Such incidences, which are rare, may indicate an important genetic health problem that needs to be monitored by a physician. If your family seems to be at particularly high risk, it is essential that you inform your children. It only makes sense for them to be aware of how important it is to start developing healthy life-style patterns early in life.

CONTROLLABLES

You can't change your age, your gender, or your ancestry, but there are several risk factors over which, fortunately, you do have some control. If you've had a heart attack, chances are that one, or more likely several, of these risk factors apply to you.

Smoking

If you smoke more than 10 cigarettes a day, you are doubling your risk of heart attack. Why are cigarettes so dangerous? Let me count the ways.

One of the most detrimental elements is the nicotine they contain. This chemical stimulates your adrenal glands, which produce adrenaline, which speeds up your heart rate and increases your blood pressure. Smoking even one or two cigarettes sometimes causes an increase of 15 to 25 beats per minute (from 75 to 95) in the heart rate. Nicotine also causes your blood vessels to constrict, thereby making your heart work harder to pump blood through your system, and it attaches itself to platelets in the blood, causing excess clotting in the arteries and veins. Finally, there is evidence that nicotine interferes with the liver's disposal of certain fats, thereby causing more fat to collect in your arteries. Inhaling cigarette smoke also increases the carbon monoxide level in your blood and decreases the oxygen count. Since less oxygen is being distributed by the blood, your heart must work even harder to keep the body adequately supplied.

Now practically everyone knows that cigarette smoking is horribly dangerous, but knowing and acting on that knowledge are two different things. I've even had patients try to sneak a smoke in the cardiac care unit. We've found cigarettes hidden under mattresses and inside pillowcases. Perhaps the most crafty patient I've encountered was a man who hid cigarettes in the urinal. Despite their attempts to get around the rules, heart patients are forced to give up cigarette smoking in the CCU, since it's forbidden around the unit's highly inflammable oxygen machines. Some resume the habit as soon as they can, despite the fact that they've received the strongest warning their bodies can give them.

I don't mean to sound unsympathetic; we all know it is not easy to quit smoking, especially if you have been doing it for years. One way to start your antismoking effort is with some self-analysis. Psychiatrists believe there are four types of smokers:

- **Addictive smokers.** These people are addicted to the nicotine rush they get when they light up. They smoke for the temporary "smoker's high."
- **Inattentive smokers.** They like the feel of a cigarette between their fingers. Many light a cigarette, play with it a bit, and then let it burn down in the ashtray.

- **Diversion smokers.** They like to watch the smoke rise. Like inattentive smokers, they play with their cigarettes more than they smoke them, but for them the attraction is visual. If they're in a dark room where they can't watch the smoke curl, they have no desire to smoke.
- **Oral smokers.** They crave what psychiatrists call "oral gratification." That is, they like having something in or near their mouths. For them, a cigarette betwen the lips is a comfort in itself.

Did you spot yourself as one or more of the "types" listed above? Once you find your type, you should have a better understanding of how you might be able to stop. For example, if you're an oral smoker, think of something else you can use for oral gratification. A stick of gum or celery may do the trick. If you're an inattentive smoker, try handling a pencil or paper clips instead of a cigarette. Diversion smokers may find it helpful to do exercises at their desks the next time they get bored. Addictive smokers may want to ask their doctors about special nicotine-flavored gums or other prescriptions that might help curb nicotine cravings. When in doubt, try all these strategies. They can't hurt, and they may help.

Here are a few more tips for smokers who are trying to call it quits:

- If your spouse is a smoker, try to convince him or her to join you in your antismoking campaign.
- Tell your family and friends you are trying to quit. This will put pressure on you to follow through.
- Don't drink alcohol to excess; most smokers report they want to smoke when they're drinking.
- Don't carry cigarettes.
- Keep a supply of gum, mints, or breath spray handy.

- Don't go out to the theater lobby during intermission.
- Sit in the no-smoking sections of restaurants planes and trains.
- When you feel the urge to nibble, try nibbling such low-calorie vegetables as celery and carrots.
- Drink lots of water.
- If you're cutting down instead of quitting "cold turkey," don't buy cigarettes by the carton. Make it a chore to go out and buy every pack.
- Start smoking a brand of cigarettes you don't like; if you detest menthol cigarettes, resolve to smoke only these.
- Remember that quitting smoking is the best thing you can do for yourself. Notice that you're sleeping better, coughing less, and regaining your sense of taste and smell. Your breath is sweeter, your clothes smell fresher, and you have a little more disposable income.
- Don't be tempted to pick up another cigarette after quitting. Most ex-smokers cannot have just one without falling back into the same old habit.

Of course, you don't have to quit smoking completely on your own. There are many clinics and organized groups that can help in your efforts. Basically, these clinics and groups use either aversion therapy or behavior modification. I recommend behavior modification—in my opinion Smokenders is the best—for heart patients, because it uses positive reinforcement to help you cut down slowly. A typical program will have you meeting with about 20 other smokers for several weeks.

Aversion therapy—Schick is the best example I know—is usually faster than behavior modification, but because you are taught to feel utterly repulsed by the sight of a cigarette, it can be stressful. Some people find that this method backfires: They become so anxious that they want a cigarette to relieve their anxiety!

If you would like some advice about the best way to quit, ask around. Talk to your doctor; contact the American Heart Association, the American Cancer Society, and the American Lung Association for information about support groups; look in the Yellow Pages; ask your friends how they did it. No matter how you decide to quit, however, the bottom line is that you *must* quit. Once you give up cigarettes, your risk of having another heart attack will drop dramatically, by 50 percent. And it doesn't take long for your body to begin to recover from the effects of smoking. Physicians have found that within two weeks of not smoking, the carbon monoxide level in your blood will be reduced to normal. If you go without smoking for 10 years, your heart and lungs will perform as if you never smoked at all.

Quit now. If you continue to smoke after your first heart attack, you are cutting your life expectancy in half.

Hypertension

Perhaps you know this disease by its other name, high blood pressure. Or perhaps you've heard it referred to as "the silent killer." Under any name, it is a deadly disease, and it can sneak up without any warning signs or symptoms. Fifty percent of all people with hypertension don't even know about their condition.

Blood pressure is the force that your heart exerts when it pumps blood through your arteries and veins. If this force becomes too great, the result is high blood pressure. It is not just your heart that overworks when you suffer from this condition; your arteries also experience extensive wear and tear. Eventually, these arteries may become hardened, scarred, inelastic, and therefore unable to function properly. The kidneys, too, may be harmed. Because the kidneys depend on receiving a great deal of blood for proper functioning, when the blood vessels break down because of hypertension, the result could be kidney failure.

Strokes, which result when the blood vessels in the brain are ruptured, are a frequent complication of very severe hypertension. This condition is as serious as it sounds; it may cause an intracerebral hemorrhage, a hematoma, and paralysis.

The only way to find out if you have high blood pressure is to undergo a blood pressure screening. It's a quick, simple procedure—a blood pressure cuff is wrapped around your arm and a reading is taken. If you have reason to think that you suffer from hypertension, be sure to have the test done at least three times to guarantee that the diagnosis is correct. Since blood pressure varies so much from day to day, a patient should be diagnosed as having hypertension only if the three test results show an elevated pressure. I tell my patients to steer clear of the free blood pressure screenings that are offered in drugstores and shopping malls. High blood pressure is a serious ailment. The sooner it is discovered, the sooner it can be brought under control. Don't take chances with a misdiagnosis. Have your screenings done in a physician's office.

By the way, if you are a large person, make sure the doctor or nurse uses a seven-inch cuff instead of the standard five-inch cuff. A cuff that is too small could make the reading inaccurate.

When I was in medical school, the rule of thumb for normal blood pressure was a person's age plus 100; hence a fifty-year-old man could be satisfied with a systolic reading of 150. Today we know that the figures we used were all wrong. In fact, anything over 140 is considered dangerous. If your blood pressure is 160, your chances of having a heart attack are double those of someone with normal blood pressure.

What is normal blood pressure? For an adult it's 120/80. (Elderly women are a notable exception. Many of them may have a much higher blood pressure—up to 170/95—and enjoy a normal life span. While these women are not usually treated for hypertension, they are closely watched.) The first number represents the systolic pressure (pressure in the blood vessels when the heart is pumping). The second number represents the diastolic pressure (pressure in the blood vessels when the heart relaxes). Most doctors agree that mild hypertension ranges from 140/90 to 159/94. People in this category have a 50 percent greater chance of having a heart attack than those with a normal rate.

No one is exactly sure what causes hypertension, but there are several theories: High blood pressure often runs in families, so heredity may have something to do with it; high blood pressure is more common among blacks than whites, so there may be a genetic factor; high blood pressure is more common in obese people, but some very thin people often become hypertensive.

We do know that there are ways you can control high blood pressure. Some simple measures include:

- **Losing weight.** An estimated 50 percent of all people with high blood pressure are overweight. Studies have shown that the condition sometimes disappears once a patient reaches his or her correct body weight.
- **Cutting down on salt.** Your body retains fluid from the sodium contained in salt. Because your heart has to pump around all that extra fluid, it has to work harder.
- **Taking medication.** Many doctors try to avoid prescribing medication for high blood pressure because of

the side effects (diuretics and beta blockers have been known to cause fatigue, apathy, muscle pain, and sometimes impotence), but if your doctor has recommended medication, take it regularly, as prescribed. Discontinuing your medication without your doctor's permission can be dangerous, even fatal.

- **Getting help from your family.** Ask your spouse or another family member to support you in your efforts to bring your blood pressure under control. This support may include gentle reminders to take your medicine, eat right, exercise, and stop smoking.

Diabetes

Under normal conditions, the pancreas creates insulin, a hormone that metabolizes digested sugars and carbohydrates. When the pancreas fails to do its job and stops producing insulin, you develop diabetes. Uncontrolled diabetes causes a dangerous chain of events. First, unmetabolized sugar accumulates in the blood, raising the cholesterol level. Second, that high level of cholesterol may contribute to the development of atherosclerosis in the heart, brain, and legs. Third, this blocked circulation can cause a heart attack, stroke, blindness, even the loss of a limb.

Fortunately, there are ways to keep diabetes under control so those problems will not occur. Thanks to modern medicine, diabetes is not a death sentence; in fact, most diabetics can lead normal lives, provided they get the proper treatment. In order to discuss the treatment of diabetes, we must describe the two kinds.

Type I Diabetes. Formerly called *juvenile diabetes,* Type I occurs most often in children and young adults. It usually appears abruptly and progresses rapidly. Because the pancreas produces little or no insulin, these people must take daily injections of insulin to keep their blood sugar at a normal level.

Type II Diabetes. Formerly called *maturity onset diabetes,* Type II often occurs in people more than forty years of age. This is the most common form of the disease; 90 percent of all diabetics have Type II. No one knows exactly why this condition develops, but there is some evidence that Type II diabetes may be hereditary. It also seems to strike people who are obese, inactive, and under a great deal of stress.

Type II diabetes is generally milder than Type I, and in most cases it can be controlled, sometimes even cured, without complicated medical intervention. If you have developed Type II diabetes, your doctor will probably recommend a special exercise and diet plan. Don't worry. This does not mean you will have to eat hospital food for the rest of your life. While some foods may be prohibited, you may still be permitted to eat many of the things you like, as long as you are sensible about how much you eat. You may have to lose weight as well. You will also be advised to start exercising, but the exercise will be moderate and gradual. No one expects you to become a superathlete.

As with high blood pressure, many people with Type II diabetes don't know they have it. If you suspect that you might be suffering from it, watch for these five warning signs:

1. Excessive thirst or hunger
2. Frequent need to urinate
3. Skin infections
4. Fatigue
5. Bruises that heal slowly

If you have two or more of these symptoms, call your physician. In order to give an accurate diagnosis your doctor will recommend that you undergo a urine test; unmetabolized sugar shows up in the urine. If this test is positive, you may also need a glucose tolerance test, which assesses how your body uses glucose, or blood sugars. Like a cholesterol count, this test should be performed several months after your heart attack, so that your body chemistry will have had time to return to normal.

Having diabetes doesn't make you an invalid. Remember, it is often possible to reverse the effects of Type II diabetes. Most diabetics suffering from either juvenile or adult diabetes are able to control their disease and lead normal, healthy, active lives.

Obesity

Watching your weight is essential in preventing heart disease. If you have had a heart attack, you must not become obese. If you are obese, you must lose weight.

Obesity is defined as being more than 30 percent over your normal weight (consult the chart on page 150 for your normal weight). Obesity is particularly prevalent in this country, where food is plentiful, and physical labor is largely unnecessary in most people's lives. And on top of that we are bombarded with advertisements for high-fat, high-calorie treats such as fast foods, sweets, and alcohol.

I try to explain it to my patients as simply as possible: If you are obese, you are making your heart work harder than it should. For every excess pound of fat you carry on your body, your heart has to pump through an extra three-quarters of a mile of blood vessels. If you have angina and are obese, the problems are severer still: Because those extra pounds increase the load on your already strained heart, you will feel even more pain.

As I mentioned before, the controllable risk factors tend to be related. If you are obese, your chances of having high blood pressure, an elevated cholesterol level, and diabetes are significantly greater than if you keep your weight down. If obesity is your problem, you need to lose weight. See chapter 13 for some suggestions.

Fats and Cholesterol

The relationship of diet to heart disease has created a great deal of controversy among medical experts over the past few years, and often the arguments have generated more heat than light. One thing most physicians seem to agree on is the necessity of watching your intake of saturated fats, cholesterol, and triglycerides. Fats can build up inside and narrow the arteries, resulting in atherosclerosis.

Studies have found that the traditional American way of eating has helped contribute to our country's high incidence of heart disease. Typically, 19 percent of the American diet is made up of fat. For the Japanese, who suffer far fewer heart attacks than Americans, only 3 percent of their diet is fat.

Sometimes drug therapy is recommended to reduce the amount of cholesterol in your body. However, such remedies must be carefully monitored, since the drugs may cause side effects. I'm generally opposed to these drugs; I much prefer to see my patients being careful about the foods they eat.

Caffeine

Without even knowing it, hundreds of thousands of people are actually addicted to caffeine and have been for a long time. Long before they had to start the day with a couple of cups of strong coffee, there were the colas and the chocolate bars. It's hard to believe that anything that seems to make you feel as good as those things do can possibly be bad for you.

But it's true. The American Heart Association has found that when consumed in large quantities, caffeine puts a tremendous strain on your heart. It works as an extremely strong stimulant, which increases the heart rate and blood pressure and gives you a sudden, unnatural "rush." Some experts estimate that one cup of strong coffee is equivalent to half an amphetamine tablet. Many people find that a cup of coffee three or four hours before bedtime can make it difficult for them to fall asleep.

People in perfect health can probably have a couple of cups of coffee a day, but if you've had a heart attack, you should give serious thought to eliminating caffeine from your life. Rethink that ritual morning cup of coffee or tea. If you can't quit cold turkey (caffeine withdrawal often causes headaches, but they should disappear within a week), remember that the stronger your coffee or tea is, the more caffeine it contains. Remember too that caffeine is often contained in soft drinks and chocolate desserts. Give decaffeinated coffee, caffeine-free sodas, and herbal teas a try.

Alcohol

It may seem strange, since we've all seen how animated people can become when they've had a drink or two, but alcohol is a depressant. Even a little alcohol slows the heart muscle's contracting abilities, and too much can affect it so much that it can no longer function efficiently. There is growing evidence that consuming more than three or four drinks a day may increase your chances of having a heart attack.

Alcohol consumption may be dangerous for patients recovering from very severe heart attacks. During the recovery period it's vital that the heart slowly regain its ability to work efficiently, and alcohol may well be an impediment to the healing process.

For those not completely restricted from alcohol, the American Heart Association recommends a maximum of 2 mixed drinks, 8 ounces of wine, or 12 ounces of beer each day. I try to persuade my patients to choose wine, since it has fewer calories than beer, and it doesn't need any high-calorie mixers. I warn them not to go over the limit by drinking light wine or beer. This may lead to a loss of control over your drinking patterns.

Before you make any choices about what to drink, talk the whole subject over with your doctor. Everyone reacts differently to alcohol, and while it can be very pleasant indeed to have a drink once in a while, you must be sure that you're not taking any risks with your health.

There is also some evidence (from researchers in France) that a glass of wine a day may actually protect you from coronary artery disease. These studies have gotten a great deal of press attention—I have a huge collection of clippings brought in by jubilant patients—but the studies are by no means conclusive. Experiments are still being conducted.

Drugs

There is no room for recreational drugs in cardiac rehabilitation. (I'm not here to pass moral judgment on the way you live your life; I'm only saying that drugs play havoc with your heart.) When you're trying to prevent a second heart attack, every drug that passes your lips, even an aspirin or an antacid tablet, must be prescribed or approved by your doctor.

If you're not convinced, consider the following:

- Marijuana elevates the heart rate and sometimes the blood pressure, making the muscle work overtime.
- Cocaine, PCP, and amphetamines may increase the heart rate and blood pressure to dangerous levels. Cocaine, particularly an intravenous dose, may cause cardiac failure. Even if you've tried cocaine a hundred times without ill effects, the hundred and first time can kill you.
- Barbiturates slow down the heart rate, sometimes so much that it no longer functions efficiently.
- Amyl nitrate lowers the blood pressure, dilating the arteries and veins and sending blood to the body's extremities. Your heart may become overworked by having to pump out too much blood at once.

In short, there's only one thing a recovering heart patient can do when it comes to drugs—don't use them.

Sedentary Life-style

He doesn't jog, doesn't swim, doesn't play tennis. If he needs something at the drugstore three blocks away, he takes the car. He always rides the elevator to the second floor. Sound like anyone you know? You're probably nodding your head, since most people who have had heart attacks are, to say the least, inactive. And inactivity may be hazardous to your health.

Exercise helps the heart in several ways. First, it strengthens all your muscles, including the heart muscle. The stronger your heart becomes, the less it will have to work to allow your body to function normally. Second, it burns calories and consequently helps to combat obesity. And third, exercise helps to reduce stress, since it uses up some of the adrenaline that your body needs for *fight or flight* responses. As you can see, exercise is one of the most important parts of any cardiac rehabilitation program.

Now I'm not saying that you should drop this book and dash out to take a few laps around the track. After years of inactivity your body will require a gradual introduction to physical exertion. Moderation is important to everyone, but it is vital for the heart attack patient, whose body is still recovering. The first thing you must do is have a stress test. Then you'll set realistic goals and expectations and, with the help of your doctor, plan an exercise program that fits your needs and your schedule.

Stress

Do you bite your nails? Drum your fingers across desk tops? Explode in fits of anger over seemingly minor matters? Or do you just feel anxious all the time? Perhaps you're becoming "stressed out." If prolonged, this condition can seriously damage your heart.

Every time you experience a stressful situation, your brain alerts the body to begin its fight or flight response. This means that your endocrine system immediately begins producing hormones called *adrenaline*. The adrenaline then prepares the body for action: muscles tense; blood pressure soars; the heart beats faster. Imagine what would happen if your body were to undergo a fight or flight response several times in the space of an hour or so. Obviously, you would quickly wear yourself out.

If you're recovering from a heart attack, it's very important to control the elements that bring about stress in your life. Most of the time this does not mean making major changes in your job or family life. It simply means reserving more time for relaxation.

Don't get caught up in what you've heard about "Type A" and "Type B" personalities. The theory—that the Type A individual is more prone to heart attacks than the Type B—might have made a catchy gimmick, but it has virtually nothing to do with the facts. As the theory went, the typical Type A is the individual who pressures himself to walk faster, talk faster, and have everything done quicker and more precisely than anyone else. Small irritants throw the Type A personality into a rage. The typical Type B individual is more passive, going about things more slowly and taking life's problems in stride. The problem with the theory is that it doesn't hold up.

There's practically no such thing as a pure Type A or a pure Type B. Most of us have characteristics of both. If pushed hard enough, nearly all of us will react with Type A characteristics sometimes in our lives. What worries me most about this theory is how I've seen my patients react to it. For example, one man I was treating had decided that he was a Type A, and he had an almost fatalistic attitude about it, as if he had nothing to say about how he reacted to stress.

As a heart patient you must realize that the so-called "Type A response" is not healthy. Like all the other controllable risk factors, stress is something you must work at controlling. If you don't, you're increasing your chances of having another heart attack.

11 Sex and Your Heart

A few years ago I received a mysterious telephone call from one of my patients. "I'd like to come in and talk to you about a problem I'm having," he said, almost in a whisper. When I asked him what the problem was, he said he'd rather not discuss it over the phone. We made an appointment for later in the week.

The next morning I got a call from his wife. "My husband doesn't know I'm calling you, but I wonder if I could come in and see you about something," she said. She didn't want to discuss it any further over the phone either. I asked her to come in the day after I was scheduled to see her husband.

As you've probably guessed by now, the subject that each of them wanted to talk about was sex, and what they had to say was not in the least bit unusual. My patient had been home from the hospital for four months, and while he was feeling great, he and his wife had yet to have sex. My patient seemed to have lost interest, and his wife was too nervous about his health to try to change his mind.

Their marriage was strong, and according to what they both told me, before his heart attack they had really enjoyed their sex life. There was no physical explanation for my patient's apparent loss of sex drive. What, then, was the problem?

Like many problems about sex, this one was caused by a communications breakdown. My patient was afraid that his sexual performance would be affected by the heart attack. His wife was afraid that having sex might bring on another heart attack. Both of them knew better—I had told them very specifically that there was no reason for them not to resume their normal sex life—but that didn't keep them from worrying.

However, the real problem was that they kept their fears to themselves. Fortunately, they did finally discuss their concerns with me, and I was able to persuade them to take the next step: to talk to each other openly and honestly. Once they started talking, they were able to relax, and once they were able to relax, their sex life went back to normal.

Unfortunately, not all of us feel comfortable talking about sex, even to our physicians. Many patients don't mind having their doctors care for their bodies, but they are reluctant to ask questions about this most intimate part of their lives. (They want to know about sex, but they're afraid to ask.) If you have sexual problems during your recovery from a heart attack, talk to your doctor, and be specific. If your questions are vague and nonspecific, chances are the answers will be vague and nonspecific too.

Other patients have a different reason for not wanting to discuss sex with their doctors—a fear of the restrictions the doctor will impose. The truth is, the only restrictions that a doctor usually will impose on a heart patient is to advise the patient to wait for a while after a heart attack—anywhere from two weeks to six is normal—before resuming full sexual activities. A study published in the *American Journal of*

Nursing stated that many heart patients begin reviving sexual activity by masturbating while still in the hospital.

It's not just patients who have trouble talking about sexual matters. Every once in a while you'll encounter a doctor who is reluctant to discuss sexual activity with you in a meaningful manner. If this happens to you, find another qualified health professional who is knowledgeable in both heart disease treatment and sexual counseling. Psychiatrists, psychologists, social workers, and nurses working in a cardiac care unit are often very helpful. Cardiac rehabilitation centers can also provide useful advice.

MYTHS ABOUT SEX

Whoever is counseling you on sexual relations during your recovery period will want to start by alleviating some of the most common fears experienced by heart patients and their sexual partners. These include:

- The fear that sexual intercourse will cause another heart attack or even sudden death. There is no evidence to suggest this.
- The fear that resuming sexual activity will somehow accelerate the patient's underlying heart disease. There are no such documented cases.
- The fear that your sexual activity was the cause of the heart attack in the first place. Sexual activity has nothing to do with the way your heart functions.

Most of the sexual fears and apprehensions, occasional depression, and the loss of sexual appetite you and your partner may experience after a heart attack can be dispelled through education, reassurance, and counseling. For example, if you feel you lack sexual desire because you are depressed after your heart attack, your doctor should explore the cause and work with you to treat the underlying factors that are causing the depression. It's perfectly natural to be depressed when you're recovering from a heart attack, but fortunately, these feelings go away quickly. And there's no reason it should be a permanent block to your sexual enjoyment.

RESUMING SEXUAL ACTIVITY

Most doctors will recommend resuming sexual activity with your regular partner anywhere from two to six weeks after your heart attack. However, there is no rule about this. Your doctor will make specific recommendations according to your individual needs.

Sexual Energy

You may be surprised to know the "energy cost" of sex is relatively low. During an orgasm, the average patient's heart rate goes up from approximately 80 to about 115 beats per minute, stays elevated for 15 to 30 seconds, and quickly returns to the normal resting heart rate. This is equivalent to climbing one or two flights of stairs. If you can climb a couple of flights of stairs without any ill effects, you are probably ready to resume sexual activity.

An important point to consider is that the frequency and quality of your sexual activity will usually improve during cardiac rehabilitation, since you're taking better care of yourself. If you follow a program of sensible eating and increased physical activity, your sex life should actually get better.

Specific Advice About Sex

As I said above, you should be specific when talking about your sexual concerns. Here's some advice:

1. Involve your regular partner in any sexual discussion you have with your doctor. You are both responsible for reestablishing a sexual partnership that both of you will be comfortable with, so you both need to learn about the best way to achieve your sexual goals.
2. Recognize that further heart attacks, or sudden death during intercourse, do not occur in the normal patient.
3. In general, avoid sex if you are tired or angry with your partner. The best time to have sex is when you're rested, relaxed, and in a good mood.
4. In the early stages of recovery from a heart attack, it is wise to wait an hour or two after a regular meal before having sex. Avoid sex if you are intoxicated or have eaten a heavy meal.
5. The room temperature should be as comfortable as possible. If the room is too hot, you may vasodilate; if it's too cold, you may vasoconstrict.
6. In the early stages of resuming sexual activity, avoid extramarital sex or sexual activity with a new partner. Both impose large energy costs.
7. Angina during sexual intercourse can probably be avoided by taking nitroglycerin just as you start your sexual activity. Your doctor may also recommend other medications to prevent angina.
8. The position used during sexual intercourse has no significant effect on the amount of work your heart does. The only thing that matters is that you and your partner are comfortable.
9. Masturbation, mutual masturbation, and oral sex do not appear to have a detrimental effect on the heart. The data on anal intercourse are not conclusive, so it should be undertaken with a greater degree of caution.
10. Only 10 percent of all heart attack patients will have problems with impotence, premature ejaculation, or failure to reach previously attainable orgasms. If any of these occurs, discuss it with your doctor. Sometimes the problem is caused by the medication you're taking. If the

problem is psychological in origin, your doctor may suggest that you consult a counselor who specializes in sexual relations.

A True Story

A couple concerned about resuming their sex life after the husband's heart attack came into my office one day to talk. As the wife explained, ever since her husband's heart attack, he had claimed to be impotent and refused even to attempt to engage in sexual activity with her.

I couldn't understand why the heart attack had affected my patient's sexual potency—I hadn't prescribed any medication—so I suggested that he take a few tests. After studying the results, I was even more puzzled. I said to my patient, who was well into his fifties, "You're about as potent as a twenty-year-old. I can't understand why you think the heart attack has made you impotent."

He sheepishly admitted the truth. After his heart attack, he'd taken up with two other women. Sheer exhaustion had left him unable to perform while with his wife.

As this story illustrates, your heart attack should not hamper your sexual appetite or your activity. Of course, I'm not saying the attack will increase it. The man with the two new women friends was an unusual case, but be assured that when it comes to sex, very little will change after your recovery.

12

Food and Your Heart

What has 51 grams of fat, 114 milligrams of cholesterol, 1,404 milligrams of sodium, and 1,116 calories? It's one of America's favorite meals—a large burger, french fries, and a chocolate shake.

And that's just the beginning. Many of the foods we routinely indulge in are true nutritional disasters. For example, there are between 800 and 900 calories in a take-out fried chicken dinner. Ten ounces of chili from a fast-food stand may have as much as 1,100 milligrams of sodium. The quarter-pound burger with cheese has a whopping 90 grams of cholesterol packed between its buns.

The sad fact is that even though maintaining a healthy diet is important in preventing heart disease, most of us have always considered the convenience, flavor, and cost of food before thinking about its nutritional value. Check your kitchen cabinets. If you are like most people, you'll find potato chips, soda pop, canned soups, canned fruits, packaged cookies, and pancake mix lurking in there somewhere.

But that's all behind you now. Your doctor has probably told you to lose weight (more about that in chapter 13), but perhaps even more significantly, you have learned that there are certain foods you should avoid and certain others you should incorporate into your daily diet. You have been told in no uncertain terms that if you're going to get well and live a long, productive life, you'll need to learn a little something about nutrition, and that is what this chapter is all about. As you read it, keep in mind that the information here is only an introduction to the subject. Read other books and articles on the subject (see the recommended reading list at the back of this book). Talk about it with your doctor and other professionals in the field. They'll be able to make some additional recommendations tailored especially for your needs.

BASIC NUTRITION

You need food to live. Your body depends on food for life-sustaining nutrients, without which it would not have the chemicals or energy necessary for the basic functions of life, such as the formation of new tissue cells, blood flow, and the transmission of brain impulses. There are certain nutrients that the body uses in particularly large quantities: fats, carbohydrates, and proteins. Water is essential. Other nutrients, such as minerals and vitamins, are important for staying alive and healthy. Each kind of nutrient provides a unique type of life-preserving chemical; you cannot survive without any one of them. The key to a good diet is to maintain a balance among the types of nutrients you consume.

CALORIES

The energy provided by the nutrients is measured in units called *calories*. As we all know, calories are associated with weight gain; when you consume too many nutrients, your body cannot use all the energy provided. It stores the excess calories as fat. Each nutrient provides different levels of calories for the body. Fat provides 9 calories per gram; carbohydrates provide 5; and protein, 4. There are approximately 3,500 calories in a pound of fat.

PROTEIN

Many people regard protein as a "power food." We've all heard of athletes who load up on steak the night before a big game. In truth, protein need only make up 15 to 20 percent of your daily calories. Your body depends on protein to supply it with amino acids—which help repair tissue cells in addition to replacing enzymes, hormones, and antibodies—but there is no need to load up on protein-rich foods. Some of the proteins you need can even be synthesized by your body.

The protein source that probably comes to mind most quickly is beef, but there are many better sources of this nutrient, since 60 percent of the calories in beef come from fat. Other, relatively low-fat sources of protein are poultry, fish, nonfat dairy products, beans and other legumes, grains, nuts, and seeds. That athlete would be better off with a plate of spaghetti. Or he could take a lesson from Chinese cooks; using small amounts of meat to flavor your meals saves calories, cuts down on fat, and saves money.

CARBOHYDRATES

Carbohydrates are the major source of your body's energy. In fact, 44 percent of the average American's diet comes from carbohydrates (as compared to 42 percent from fat and 14 percent from protein). Experts say that in a healthy diet that number should be closer to 60 percent.

But that doesn't mean you can rush right out and start eating doughnuts. No, the carbohydrates that nutritionists are so keen on are complex carbohydrates, the fibers and starches that burn slowly, aid digestion, and provide a steady source of energy. The most nutritious of the complex carbohydrates are vegetables, fruits, legumes, nuts, seeds, whole grains, pasta, and rice. No doughnuts.

Doughnuts are simple carbohydrates, or sugars, which burn quickly and are converted to glucose. They do not aid in digestion; in fact, they tend to load the body with excess energy, which is converted to fat. Sugar also raises the body's insulin and triglyceride levels, eventually causing light-headedness, weakness, and fatigue.

You should watch your sugar intake, but don't think that just means putting away the sugar bowl. Processed foods are filled with sugar. And by the way, you aren't doing yourself a favor by substituting honey for sugar; honey is about 75 percent sugar. Despite some claims that it is "more natural" than table sugar, the fact is that honey is no better than what you have in your sugar bowl right now.

FATS

Fats are essential for maintaining the body's structure and providing insulation for body heat. They transport certain vitamins throughout the body; without them, severe vitamin deficiencies can result. Fats are a wonderful energy source. They're even good for the skin. Why, then, are they public enemy number one? First, because they make us fat, which makes us vulnerable to heart problems. Second, because—according to many scientists—they clog the arteries and make blood distribution throughout the system very difficult. This condition often causes atherosclerosis, which may lead to a heart attack.

Just as there are two kinds of carbohydrates, there are two major kinds of fats: saturated and unsaturated. Saturated fats, which are found in animal products and some vegetable products (coconut and palm oil especially), should be avoided as much as possible. They are the ones that clog your arteries. Unsaturated fats are the oils from vegetable products, such as safflowers, sunflowers, corn, soybeans, cottonseeds, peanuts, and olives. They appear to have a beneficial effect on the heart.

Unsaturated fats also fall into two categories: monounsaturated fats, which do not seem to have much effect on the body's fat levels; and polyunsaturated fats, which appear to help in proper fat distribution, thus preventing its dangerous accumulation in the body.

According to the American Heart Association, a healthy diet includes less than 30 percent fat. Some health professionals say that 20 percent is plenty. To be on the safe side, a recovering heart patient should probably split the difference. I tell my patients to aim for 25 percent. Start by cutting down on red meat, butter, cheese, and mayonnaise. Avoid packaged foods of any kind and stay out of fast food restaurants. Learn the nomenclature; you should know, for instance, that while "hydrogenated oil" may *sound* healthy, it means saturated fat.

Choose lean cuts of meat, skinless chicken and fish, and nonfat and low-fat dairy products. Low-fat and nonfat yogurt, cottage cheese, and milk are available in just about every grocery store these days. If you are used to whole milk and regular cheeses, these products may take a little getting used to, but thinking about your clear, healthy arteries may help you acquire a taste for them.

CHOLESTEROL AND TRIGLYCERIDES

Cholesterol and triglycerides are incredibly popular subjects with the media today. You can barely pick up a newspaper or a magazine without being bombarded with the latest findings. The problem is that what you read this morning tends to contradict what you read yesterday. Such information makes some people obsessed with cholesterol. I've seen patients who have a blood cholesterol reading done every week. Patients should remember that there is a great deal of variation in these measurements.

Let's cover the basics. Cholesterol and triglycerides are fatty substances called *lipids,* which may contribute to the buildup of fatty deposits in your system. Eighty-five percent of the cholesterol in your blood is manufactured by your liver; only 15 percent is absorbed through the foods you eat. Therefore, if you are asked to change your diet to reduce your cholesterol intake, you are actually affecting only a small percent of your total cholesterol level. The rest increases or decreases depending on your natural body chemistry. (The same is true for triglycerides. Much of this substance is also made in the body and has no bearing on how much or how little you consume.)

There are two types of cholesterol: LDL, or low-density lipoprotein, cholesterol is believed to be the "bad" type. It occurs when cholesterol is linked to your consumption of saturated fat. LDL joins with the triglycerides in your blood to leave fatty deposits in the arteries. Then there is HDL, or high-density lipoprotein, the "good" cholesterol. HDL is linked to your consumption of polyunsaturated fats, and its major function is joining with triglycerides to deliver fat products to the liver and other body sites for metabolization or elimination.

Most people consume about 400 to 450 milligrams of cholesterol per day. For the person trying to stick to a low-cholesterol diet, only about 300 daily milligrams of cholesterol should be consumed. If your doctor has indicated that your blood cholesterol level is abnormally high (above 220 milligrams), he or she may recommend that you stay away from foods that are naturally high in cholesterol. Don't panic. You will not be condemned to a diet of parsley and carrots for the rest of your life.

Some very common sources of cholesterol are meat, shellfish, egg yolks, liver, organ meats, and butterfat. You'll notice that all of these foods come from animals. Foods from plants do not have cholesterol, although they may contain saturated fat. When you are following a low-cholesterol, low-triglyceride, and low-saturated fat regimen, your best bet is to eat fish (not shellfish), vegetables, fruit, plain breads, and cereals. Make substitutions in cooking: egg whites instead of whole eggs; low-fat or nonfat yogurt instead of sour cream; and margarine in place of butter (make sure the oil in your margarine is not hydrogenated).

No discussion of cholesterol would be complete without mentioning Omega-3 fatty acids. Recent evidence suggests that the oil in cold-water fish (salmon, sardines, tuna, and others) may contribute to lowering the body's triglyceride and cholesterol levels. The oil in fish is very different from the fats in other animal foods, since it contains Omega-3 fatty acids, which have an additional bonus of reducing blood clots.

If your physician tests your triglyceride level and it registers too high (above 160), you will need to cut back on your intake of saturated fats (a good idea even if you don't have a serious problem). You may need to cut down on your intake of alcohol and simple sugars, since there is some evidence that triglycerides increase in the blood when too many simple carbohydrates are consumed.

WATER

We need water as much as we need air. It cools us, aids our circulation (very important for the heart patient), and fuels our muscles. I recommend that my patients drink six glasses of water a day. If you're worried about retaining fluid, a common side effect of the medication you may be taking or of some heart ailments themselves, there is no reason for concern. Strangely enough, drinking water has nothing to do with retaining fluid. In fact, drinking water may decrease your chances of becoming bloated. Any water will do, by the way. Tap water is just as good for your heart as designer mineral water.

SALT

Salt, which technically belongs with "Minerals," below, deserves its own subhead because keeping track of salt intake is particularly important for heart patients. Many physicians have linked sodium to hypertension, an extremely serious risk factor for those with heart disease.

Your body needs sodium for proper functioning, but it doesn't need nearly so much as most of us eat. A healthy body needs only about 2,000 milligrams of salt per day, which isn't very much when you consider that there are about 1,500 milligrams in a cup of tomato sauce. In the body, excess sodium acts like a sponge, soaking up extra fluids from body tissue, and as a result, less fluid is available for blood production. When less blood is available, the heart has to work harder to supply the body with essential oxygen.

Unfortunately, you can't cut down on salt simply by removing the salt shaker from the table. It is everywhere, in virtually everything we eat. The only way to reduce your sodium intake is to be aware of what those particular high-sodium foods are. Many of our favorite foods, such as cheese, crackers, cold cuts, and pickles, are loaded with sodium. Fast food is one of the worst offenders (according to the Center for Science in the Public Interest, there is more sodium in a fast-food milkshake than there is in the french fries!), and processed foods of all kinds are just as bad.

If you cannot live without added salt, ask your doctor about using potassium chloride, a salt substitute. Better yet, try "seasoning" your food with lemon juice, vinegar, and other seasonings, such as dill, thyme, parsley, basil, sage, tarragon, chives, and oregano. They are generally safe for a salt-restricted diet.

OTHER MINERALS

Minerals are considered micronutrients for the body. That is, you do not need as many of them in your daily diet as the macronutrients—fats, carbohydrates, and proteins. However, some minerals do play essential roles in keeping your body fit. The most important are calcium, phosphorus, magnesium, iron, sodium, and potassium.

- **Calcium and phosphorus.** These are important for building and repairing bone. They are found primarily in milk (nonfat or whole) and other dairy products. Spinach, green vegetables, and beans also are good sources. Heart patients should get about 800 milligrams of phosphorus and the same amount of calcium (about two glasses of milk) per day.
- **Magnesium.** Magnesium is necessary for the conduction of nerve impulses and maintenance of cells and enzymes. Men need about 350 milligrams of magnesium in their diet, and women need about 300 milligrams. It is found in whole-grain cereals, milk, shellfish, fish, meat, fruit, vegetables, and nuts.

- **Iron.** This is essential for hemoglobin in the red blood cells. Studies show that both men and women may become anemic (iron-deficient) as they get older. Your best defense is eating such iron-rich foods as sardines, nuts, dried beans, eggs, prunes, raisins, leafy green vegetables, enriched breads, and cereals. If you are still not meeting your daily iron needs (about 18 milligrams), your doctor may suggest taking iron supplements.
- **Potassium.** This mineral is essential for maintaining the chemical balance of cellular fluids as well as ensuring heart and other muscle functioning. Good potassium sources are leafy green vegetables, tomatoes, dried fruits, bananas, potatoes, oranges, peas, beans, meats, and fish. If you are taking diuretic drugs, you may have a problem with potassium loss. If it is critical, your doctor may recommend a potassium supplement.

VITAMINS

Imagine that you could forget everything you've read in this chapter and simply take a vitamin pill that would guarantee proper nutrition. It sounds wonderful, but unfortunately it isn't possible. No matter what you may hear, a pill, no matter how strong, won't guarantee that you're getting all the nutrients you need.

Most vitamin pills pass right through your body and are eliminated during urination. As a result, you end up wasting a lot of money. Also certain vitamins can be harmful if taken in large quantities. It's just not possible for a pill to provide you with as much nutrition as a well-balanced diet, not to mention the bulk your body needs to eliminate waste products. The only way you can be sure that you're getting the proper vitamins is to eat the right foods (see the vitamin guide in this chapter for specifics). If you think you need a vitamin supplement of any kind, check with your doctor. Among other things, he'll want to be sure that a vitamin won't interfere with any of the medication you're taking.

And now for a word or two about vitamin C. There has been a lot of talk about the curative powers of vitamin C, but the vote is definitely not in yet. There is no proof that it cures or prevents colds. We do know that vitamin C helps hold body cells together, strengthens blood vessels, heals wounds, and aids in resistance to infection. On the other hand, research has shown that excess vitamin C may be associated with kidney stones and severe diarrhea. Perhaps most important for a heart patient is that too much vitamin C in the urine makes it virtually impossible to test accurately for diabetes. Unless your physician specifically tells you to take a vitamin C supplement, don't do it.

No, I'm afraid that the "miracle" of your recovery will come not from a pill but from your own efforts. All other solutions are simply fantasies.

THE LOW-FAT, LOW-CHOLESTEROL, AND LOW-TRIGLYCERIDE DIET

Eat These	*Avoid These*
Dairy	
Low-fat or nonfat milk (preferably less than 1% butterfat)	Whole milk
Evaporated low-fat or nonfat milk	Regular evaporated and dry milk
Low-fat or nonfat dry milk	
Cheese made from nonfat or low-fat milk, such as cottage cheese, farmer's, hoop, and mozzarella	All cheeses made with whole milk or cream

Nondairy creamers made from polyunsaturated fats	Nondairy creamers
Low-calorie hot cocoa	Chocolate milk
Low-fat or nonfat yogurt	Frozen yogurt from whole milk
Egg whites	Egg yolks

Breads and Starches

White enriched bread, whole wheat, rye, pumpernickel, english muffins, matzo, biscuits, Italian and French breads, raisin bread, hamburger buns, pita bread, and muffins (made with polyunsaturated oil)	Bagels made with eggs or cheese, buttery rolls, cheese breads, commercial doughnuts, muffins, sweet rolls, croissants, and waffles
Oatmeal, ready-to-eat cereals	Granola cereals with coconut or coconut oil
Rice, noodles, spaghetti, macaroni	Potato chips
Animal crackers, bread sticks, graham crackers, melba toast, saltines,* oyster crackers,* flatbread, pretzels,* and unbuttered popcorn	Cheese crackers, butter crackers, and those made with coconut or palm

Meat, Poultry, and Seafoods

Beef: Lean, well-trimmed beef (but not for more than 5 meals per week)	Prime cuts or heavily marbled meats, all untrimmed cuts, beef sausage, brisket, chili,

* High salt content—be careful!

	corned beef, ground meat, pastrami, ribs (short or spare), rib eye roast or steak
Veal: Lean, well-trimmed veal (no more than 5 meals per week)	Breast riblets
Pork: Lean, well-trimmed pork (no more than 5 meals per week)	Boston (roast or steak), ground pork, loin back ribs, shoulder arm (roast or steak), spareribs, canned deviled ham, cured ham, pigs' feet, salt pork, sausage, smoked pork hock, smoked pork shoulder, bacon
Lamb: Lean and well-trimmed (no more than 5 meals per week)	Ground lamb and mutton
All fish (limit shellfish, since they are low in fat, but high in cholesterol)	Caviar, commercially fried fish or shellfish
Skinless chicken or turkey	Fried chicken
Rabbit, pheasant, venison	Domestic duck, goose, opossum, raccoon, venison sausage
	Bologna, canned luncheon meats, frankfurters, headcheese, salami
	Liver and organ meats

Vegetables

Dark, green, leafy vegetables	Vegetables prepared with butter or cream

White or sweet potatoes without cream or animal fat	Potatoes prepared with saturated fats such as french fries or mashed
	Potatoes with butter
	Olives and avocados

Desserts

Fresh fruits	
Syrup, honey, molasses, sugar candies, mints, marshmallows*	Chocolate, cream candies
	Cashew, macadamia, and pistachio nuts
Puddings from nonfat or low-fat milk, sherbet, ice milk, low-fat frozen yogurt	Ice cream, whipping cream, frozen yogurt made with whole milk

Beverages

Herb tea, decaffeinated coffee, wine, beer, spirits (if permitted by your physician), low-calorie soda (avoid those with caffeine), skim milk and drinks made with skim milk products	Milkshakes, malts, eggnogs

Cooking Fats, Oils, and Dressings

Margarine listing liquid safflower, corn, or sunflower oil as the primary ingredient, diet margarine listing corn, safflower, or sunflower oil as the primary ingredient	Margarine not listing liquid oil as the primary ingredient, bacon, butter, chocolate, coconut, coconut oil, palm or palm kernel

* No cholesterol but extremely high in sugar and of little nutritive value—best to avoid.

Sunflower, safflower, corn, soybean, and cottonseed oil	Gravy from meat drippings, ham hocks, meat fat, suet and shortening
Low-fat mayonnaise	Regular mayonnaise
Low-calorie salad dressings, dressings made from liquid oils	Blue cheese, green goddess, roquefort, dressings made with sour cream or cheese
Olive oil (use sparingly)	

TIPS FOR EATING OUT ON A LOW-FAT, LOW-CHOLESTEROL, AND LOW-TRIGLYCERIDE DIET

Eat These:	*Avoid These:*
Italian	
Antipasti with roasted peppers, grilled vegetables, raw mushrooms, any green salad	
Pastas with marinara sauce, red or white clam sauce, oil and garlic, broccoli	Pastas stuffed with whole-milk cheeses and fatty meats or tomato sauces with prosciutto or pancetta (bacon)
Fish or seafood brodetto, Livornese, posillipo, or marechiare Cold seafood salads	
Water-based ices Fruit or fruit cooked in wine	Custards and ice creams, milk-based sherbets
French	
Mussels (steamed or grilled marinière)	Nouvelle dishes that may seem light but can have calorie-laden sauces

Vegetables à la grecque (prepared with olive oil and lemon)	Anything cooked with butter or heavy cream sauces
Snails	
Frogs' legs Provençal (sautéed in olive oil and garlic)	
Dover sole (without cream sauce)	
Stewed chicken Marengo (chicken with tomatoes, mushrooms, and white wine)	
Chicken à la diable (chicken deviled and grilled)	
Fruit soufflé made only with egg whites	Eclairs, custard, ice cream

Chinese

Hot and sour soup (without meat)	
Steamed shrimp Scallops	Cantonese sauces with eggs (traditional on fish and lobster)
Vegetables, bean curd, Szechwan cabbage	Fried rice
Chicken or fish cooked in black bean sauce	Fish or chicken dishes laced with ham

Mexican

All hot and mild relish sauces	Authentic dishes cooked in lard (ask if the chef uses vegetable oil)

Fish cooked Veracruzano (baked with red and green chili peppers)	
Arroz con pollo (chicken and rice)	
Guacamole and refried beans in moderation	

Indian

Poori, chapati, and roti breads	Anything cooked with ghee (clarified butter)
Tandoori roasted seafood or chicken	Appetizers (too hard to determine the ingredients)
Yogurt dressings, lentil sauces	

Japanese

Sushi and sashimi	Stay away from fried dishes
Anything beginning or ending with *nabe* (means cooked in broth)	
Fish and chicken in a *domburi* (means steamed with vegetables and rice or noodles)	

Note: Be careful to stick with broiled fish or chicken at Middle European, German, Russian, and American steakhouse restaurants, where foods tend to be high in cholesterol.

VITAMIN GUIDE

Vitamin A

For formation of skin, bones, and teeth; also enhances night and color vision.

Sources: liver, fish liver oils, butter and margarine, cream, specially enriched low-fat milks and cheeses, carrots, dark green leafy vegetables.

Vitamin B_1 (Thiamine)

Helps in carbohydrate metabolism.

Sources: whole-grain flours and cereals, wheat germ, sunflower and sesame seeds, peanuts, pine nuts, legumes (soybeans), organ meats, pork, leafy vegetables.

Vitamin B_2 (Riboflavin)

Helps in metabolism of carbohydrates, proteins, and fat.

Sources: liver, kidneys, cheese, milk, eggs, leafy vegetables, enriched bread, lean meat, beans, and peas.

Vitamin B_6

Involved in the metabolism of protein.

Sources: sunflower seeds, wheat germ and bran, whole-grain bread, flours and cereals, liver, meats, fish and poultry, potatoes, beans, and brown rice.

Vitamin B_{12}

Necessary for red blood cell formation and the nervous system.

Sources (animal products only): liver, meats, eggs, poultry, shellfish, and fish.

Vitamin C

Important for formation of collagen (skin's connective tissue), tendons, bone, and hemoglobin; also helps with absorption of iron and may assist with metabolism.

Sources: peppers, broccoli, cauliflower, fresh potatoes, green leafy vegetables, citrus fruits, tomatoes, cantaloupes, and other melons.

Vitamin D

Regulates intestinal absorption of calcium and phosphorus; also helps with use of these minerals in bones and soft tissues; some role in protein metabolism.

Sources: sunlight, fortified milk, fish liver oils, butter, egg yolk, liver, fatty fish such as sardines, tuna, and salmon.

Vitamin E

Prevents oxidization of Vitamin A; preserves red blood cells.

Sources: vegetable oils (cottonseed, safflower, and sunflower), corn, almonds, peanuts, wheat germ, rice germ, asparagus, green leafy vegetables, liver, margarine, and vegetable shortening.

Vitamin K

Needed for blood clotting.

Sources: usually produced by bacteria in the intestine; if a serious shortage is present, you can get it from green leafy vegetables, cauliflower, cabbage, liver, egg yolk, and soybean oil.

13

How to Lose Weight

When asked how heart surgery had changed his life, cartoonist Charles Schultz hesitated for a moment. At first the creator of *Peanuts* said that relatively little had been altered. Finally, he admitted, somewhat sheepishly, "Well, I *do* miss those marshmallow sundaes."

If you've had a heart attack, the chances are very good that your doctor has told you to lose weight. Thirty percent of all heart attack victims are overweight, and it's well known that obesity increases your chances of developing hypertension and atherosclerosis. The sooner you lose weight, the sooner you will recover from your heart attack and regain your health.

In chapter 12, I gave you a crash course in nutrition. In this chapter I'm going to try to help you stay on your diet. Even if you are not on a weight loss diet, the information here will teach you some eating habits that may prolong your life. It's true that you may not be able to have a marshmallow sundae every day, but in the long run, you'll have something much better.

WHY WE GAIN WEIGHT

"I've got a glandular problem." "I can't live without chocolate." "Dieting doesn't work for me."

How many of these things have you heard people say? How many times have you said them yourself? There is no end to the excuses we have for putting on weight. However, very few overweight patients actually have glandular problems, and we know that while it may be difficult, it's not impossible to live without certain foods, even chocolate. And as countless success stories reveal, dieting does work, if it's the *right* kind of dieting. In truth, the cause of being overweight is very simple indeed. If you consume more calories than your body needs for fuel, the excess will be stored as fat.

The main problem with obesity is that it is much easier to gain weight than to lose it. One pound of body fat contains 3,500 stored calories, which means that in order to lose a pound a week by dieting alone, you would have to decrease your caloric intake by 500 calories a day. Since most of us eat between 1,500 and 2,500 calories a day, this is quite a bit to forfeit. Once you begin to think about those numbers, it's easy to see why exercise plays such an important part in weight loss; if you burn up 250 extra calories a day and eat 250 calories fewer, you can still lose that pound a week.

FAD DIETS

"Lose 20 pounds in 20 days without feeling hungry!" It's hard not to be tempted by such a promise, even if you know that it can't be true. Every day we're virtually bombarded with promises of miracle weight loss through special diets. These diets are special, all right. Most are notorious for abusing the body with poor nutrition, virtual starvation, or even harmful drugs. They also do not teach good eating habits. Once you drop the weight as a result of a fad diet, you will bounce right back to the same unhealthy way you were eating before. As enticing as they may seem, fad diets are irrational, unsound, and unsafe, especially for those gradually gaining back their health after a heart attack.

Generally, there are several ways to determine whether or not a diet is a fad, but the most useful one is common sense. Any diet that recommends abnormal eating habits, such as consuming only fruit or powders for weeks on end or only eating one category of food or fasting, is not a normal way of eating. Beware too of the nonprescription "diet aids" that are flooding the market now. Most contain caffeine, which has been linked to an increased risk of coronary artery disease. Never take such medications while recovering from heart problems unless your doctor says it's all right.

Your best bet is to skip the fads and take another look at a medically approved diet. Better yet work out an eating plan with your doctor or nutritionist. True, these diets may not be particularly trendy or glamorous, but they are medically sound and nutritionally beneficial. Most important, they focus on what is really necessary in losing weight: forming sensible eating habits.

THE BEST DIET PROGRAM

After 25 years of talking to patients about losing weight and listening to the stories of their success and failure, I am convinced that the most effective way to lose weight is to follow a plan that has been designed specifically for you. The diet may come from your doctor, but more likely he or she will recommend that you consult a registered dietitian with experience in working with heart patients.

I have nothing against many standard-issue diets, provided they are sensible. I've seen more than a few success stories come out of Weight Watchers, for instance, and I have a great deal of admiration for what they do and how they do it. Still, as far as I'm concerned, there's no substitute for the personal touch. What if you really can't live without pizza or chocolate or a couple of glasses of wine in the evening? Or maybe you have to eat lunch out with a client every day. Or perhaps you're allergic to milk. There may be any number of factors that will play a part in your diet regimen. A dietitian can incorporate your tastes, schedule, and even some of your passions into your daily diet. You need a diet that's geared for *you,* not the other way around.

SETTING GOALS

When you set about to lose weight, you need to take time to consider your actions and then set realistic goals. First look at the "ideal weight" chart on page 150. A lot of overweight people assume that they don't fit the specifications because they're heavy-boned, but few people truly are, unless they're on the scrimmage line of the Dallas Cowboys. Study the chart and then talk to your doctor about what you should weigh. When you do set goals, don't target your weight loss to a birthday, a vacation, or any other special event. This kind of goal focuses on losing weight for the short term. You are going for weight reduction and control that will last long after Christmas.

You can expect to lose about a pound (or less) a week when you first start. It may seem agonizingly slow, but it's far healthier than dropping five pounds in just a few days. And your good health is what this diet is all about.

SHOPPING, MEAL PLANNING, AND COOKING

Dieting doesn't just involve willpower. It also involves careful planning, shopping, and food preparation. Entire books have been written about behavior modification and healthful cooking (for a list of recommended reading see the end of this book), and magazines and newspapers are filled with helpful hints.

I'm not going to try to compete with them here. I'll just pass along a few general bits of advice.

- Work out your meals at least 24 hours in advance. If you have a plan, you're less likely to do any "unscheduled" eating.
- If you are given a choice of "acceptable" foods, choose the ones that are easiest to prepare. Your new diet should not require a lot of extra effort, such as daily trips to out-of-the-way markets. The easier and more realistic your dieting plan is, the better your chances are of sticking to it.
- Make a shopping list and follow it to the letter. Eat before going shopping. If you go to the store hungry, you are more likely to buy the wrong foods.
- Avoid temptation. Don't buy or keep foods you shouldn't eat in the house. If you need snacks for guests, buy them just before they're needed and give away the leftovers. When you have finished eating, put the food away immediately. Out of sight, out of mind.
- Read labels. Most food products now have calories and other nutritional information written somewhere on the package. Don't be fooled by ambiguous wording. For example, if the label says "vegetable oil," it may well mean palm or coconut oil, which is loaded with saturated fat. Put what you learned from chapter 12 to good use.
- If you prepare meals, it may help to do your cooking when you're self-control is highest. If you can manage it, after you've finished dinner, prepare the next evening's meal.
- Make only enough food for one serving. If that doesn't make sense, dole out the portion you are meant to have and freeze the rest right away.

- Always have raw vegetables cleaned and cut and ready to nibble on. Store a platter of celery and carrots in the refrigerator so it's there when you have the irresistible urge to eat.
- Choose a specific place in one room of your home and designate this as the only place you will eat. Get out of the habit of eating in front of the TV, in the car, or in bed. When you're at work, don't eat lunch at your desk, or you may begin to associate sitting at your desk with eating.
- Do not feel you have to clean your plate. This sense of duty may be a carryover from childhood, when you were told that all good boys and girls ate what they were served. If you are a member of the "clean plate club," serve meals on smaller plates.
- Instead of placing serving bowls on the table at mealtime, put the bowls in the kitchen and serve from there. This way you will be less tempted to have seconds.
- If you are permitted to have alcohol, avoid drinking before meals. Alcohol, an appetite stimulant, tends to leave you craving sugar at the meal's end. Have your glass of wine with dinner or even afterward, as "dessert."
- Stay busy. Get involved in family projects or community activities. Many people eat out of boredom.
- Brush your teeth after each meal. Without the taste of food in your mouth, you will focus on other things.

SOCIAL OCCASIONS

Holiday and social occasions are joyous times, and they can be a great source of pleasure. They can also wreck your diet. These few tricks may help you get through them, but if you really feel you can't help overeating during social events, your doctor may suggest that you avoid them for a while.

- Have a filling snack (I recommend a small bowl of cereal or an English muffin) before you leave for the party. You'll be less likely to eat when you get there.
- Look around the table and find the thinnest person there. Match your eating speed with his or hers.
- Stick to broiled or roasted foods when eating out and ask for sauces and dressings to be placed on the side. If you regularly have lunch or dinner in the same restaurant, get to know the waiter or waitress. Ask for help in selecting the lightest meals on the menu.

WHEN YOU SLIP

Sometimes, despite the most vigorous efforts, you will slip and eat what you know is bad for you, but don't give up. Remember that this diet is not a matter of squeezing into a new pair of slacks or looking good at your class reunion. For heart patients losing weight is a matter of life and death. But because you are not a robot, you can't be programmed to change the habits of a lifetime overnight. When you get off the track, forget about it and get back on.

SUPPORT SYSTEMS

Weight loss is tough, and everyone needs a little support now and then. Here are some ways to build your own support system:

- Find somebody to diet and take walks with you. Talk about the problems you're having. Celebrate the victories.
- Remind family and friends that you need praise for even small efforts. Most people are shy about congrat-

ulating someone for not eating. Tell people that sometimes you need encouragement.

- If people tempt you with food or leave it out where it disturbs you, assert your rights. Tell them that such behavior makes it harder for you to stick to your diet.
- Check with your doctor about joining an organized support group, such as Weight Watchers or Overeaters Anonymous. Both organizations have helped many people lose weight.

EXERCISE

To be effective, dieting must be matched by a gradual increase in activity. During your convalescence and conditioning phases you will be following a structured program of exercise, but if you're tempted to taper off once you reach maintenance, think twice. Exercise plays an immensely important part in weight control. It burns calories, and there is much evidence to suggest that over a period of time it can speed up your metabolism, so that you're burning more calories even when you are at rest. In addition to the advice in chapters 9 and 14 here are a few more pointers that should help you with your exercise program.

- Always be on the lookout for opportunities to walk. Let the bus drop you off a stop or two before your usual point of departure. If your doctor says it's all right, use the stairs instead of escalators and elevators.
- Get rid of the "objects of convenience" that make you sedentary. Do you really need a remote control on our television or VCR?
- Vacuum the house twice a week instead of only once (if your doctor approves).

- If you are hungry, take a walk. Exercise often makes the hunger pangs go away.
- Don't try to trade off exercise for calories. It takes hours of exercise to burn off one chocolate doughnut.

HOW I KICKED THE ICE-CREAM HABIT

Like Charles Schultz, I have always had a weakness for ice cream. For most of my adult life I had at least a scoop or two of vanilla or strawberry every day. When my weight began to creep up bit by bit, I finally woke up to the fact that I was truly hooked on the stuff. I tried to cut down, but it didn't work. I liked it too much to have just a taste. It was obvious that I had to kick the habit completely.

I knew that aversion therapy can be used effectively to help people quit smoking, so I thought that a variation on this theme might work for me. I went out and bought the flavor of ice cream I absolutely detested: pistachio. I'm a little ashamed to say that as much as I hated pistachio, I served myself up a bowl from time to time, but that's about as far as I went. Once I tasted it, I was completely put off. In the end I decided that if it was going to be pistachio or nothing, I would choose nothing. And I did.

But don't feel sorry for me, or for Charles Schultz, or for yourself. Life without marshmallow sundaes is not that bad. In fact, it can be great

• • •

1983 METROPOLITAN HEIGHT AND WEIGHT TABLES

Height	Small Frame	Medium Frame	Large Frame
		Men	
5′ 2″	128–134	131–141	138–150
5′ 3″	130–136	133–143	140–153
5′ 4″	132–138	135–145	142–156
5′ 5″	134–140	137–148	144–160
5′ 6″	136–142	139–151	146–164
5′ 7″	138–145	142–154	149–168
5′ 8″	140–148	145–157	152–172
5′ 9″	142–151	148–160	155–176
5′ 10″	144–154	151–163	158–180
5′ 11″	146–157	154–166	161–184
6′ 0″	149–160	157–170	164–188
6′ 1″	152–164	160–174	168–192
6′ 2″	155–168	164–178	172–197
6′ 3″	158–172	167–182	176–202
6′ 4″	162–176	171–187	181–207
		Women	
4′ 10″	102–111	109–121	118–131
4′ 11″	103–113	111–123	120–134
5′ 0″	104–115	113–126	122–137
5′ 1″	106–118	115–129	125–140
5′ 2″	108–121	118–132	128–143
5′ 3″	111–124	121–135	131–147
5′ 4″	114–127	124–138	134–151
5′ 5″	117–130	127–141	137–155
5′ 6″	120–133	130–144	140–159
5′ 7″	123–136	133–147	143–163
5′ 8″	126–139	136–150	146–167
5′ 9″	129–142	139–153	149–170
5′ 10″	132–145	142–156	152–173
5′ 11″	135–148	145–159	155–176
6′ 0″	138–151	148–162	158–179

Note: Weights at ages 25–59 based on lowest mortality. Weight in pounds according to frame (in indoor clothing weighing 5 lbs. for men and 3 lbs. for women; shoes with 1-in. heels).

Source: Basic data from 1979 Build Study, Society of Actuaries and Association of Life Insurance Medical Directors of America, 1980. Courtesy of Metropolitan Life Insurance Company.

FRAME SIZE

HEIGHT IN 1″ HEELS	ELBOW BREADTH
MEN	
5′2″–5′3″	2½″–2⅞″
5′4″–5′7″	2⅝″–2⅞″
5′8″–5′11″	2¾″–3″
6′0″–6′3″	2¾″–3⅛″
6′4″	2⅞″–3¼″
WOMEN	
4′10″–4′11″	2¼″–2½″
5′0″–5′3″	2¼″–2½″
5′4″–5′7″	2⅜″–2⅝″
5′8″–5′11″	2⅜″–2⅝″
6′0″	2½″–2¾″

Source: Basic data from 1979 Build Study, Society of Actuaries and Association of Life Insurance Medical Directors of America, 1980. Courtesy of Metropolitan Life Insurance Company.

To approximate your frame size, extend your arm and bend the forearm upward at a 90-degree angle. Keep fingers straight and turn the inside of your wrist toward your body. If you have a caliper, use it to measure the space between the two prominent bones on *either* side of your elbow. Without a caliper, place thumb and index finger of your other hand on these two bones. Measure the space between your fingers against a ruler or tape measure. Compare it with these tables that list elbow measurements for *medium-framed* men and women. Measurements lower than those listed indicate you have a small frame. Higher measurements indicate a large frame.

14

The Conditioning Phase

There will come a time, usually about a month after you come home from the hospital, when you reach a turning point in your recovery. That's when the difficult convalescent phase is over, and the conditioning phase begins. For the past month or so you have been allowing your body to heal and preparing it for a new, healthy life. Now, for the next three months, you will begin to condition your body.

Your life should be getting back to normal. You've quit smoking and lost about five pounds, and you feel almost like your old self again. You're looking forward to going back to work, at least part time, and the doctor says you can start going out to dinner or seeing friends once or twice a week. You're definitely ready for conditioning.

You will be more independent and more responsible for your health during the conditioning phase. If you have been exercising in a formal cardiac rehabilitation program, your visits will continue. The important thing to remember in this conditioning phase is that you will now become more and more in charge of your own physical rehabilitation.

The conditioning phase of your recovery is, quite simply, a physical activity program through which your body gains strength and your mind gains purpose. If you were out of shape before your heart attack, you will very probably find that the program adds zest to your life. Your body will be conditioned within the limits of safety, and your goals will be realistic, but even so, you'll be surprised at what you can achieve. After a few months of conditioning many patients feel better than they've felt in years.

Remember, physical activity is one of the most important parts of your recovery program. In addition to toning your body, it will help reduce the level of cholesterol and triglycerides in your blood. Since you will be increasing your exercise performance (and, naturally, increasing the work done by your heart), it is vital that you work closely with your doctor throughout this phase. Conditioning is a progressive program, so be sure to get your doctor's approval before you move from one step to the next.

During the conditioning phase continue everything you learned during the convalescent phase: eat sensibly and adhere to your special diet, weigh yourself every day, and take a daily nap whenever you can. (If your memory is a little cloudy, go back and reread chapter 9.) If your heart attack occurred many months or even years ago, you may start your exercise program with this conditioning phase rather than the convalescent phase, but only after consulting with your doctor.

If you are engaged in a formal cardiac rehabilitation program, the number of visits that you make to the rehab center may increase during the conditioning phase. Make sure you ask the cardiac rehabilitation center staff as well as your doctor for information on this crucial turning point in your recovery.

INTRODUCING METs

When they consult with patients, nutritionists and dietitians talk a lot about calories. Cardiologists, physical therapists, and cardiac rehabilitation program staff members tend to talk about METs. No, they're not discussing the 1986 World Series; the MET they're referring to is a unit of energy expenditure. Basically, 1 MET is the amount of energy your body spends when you are at rest—sitting still or asleep, for instance. You expend 3 METs (three times the amount of energy you used when you were resting) when you clean windows or walk at a rate of 3 miles an hour; 6 METs when you shovel snow for 10 minutes; 7½ METs when you jog 5 miles an hour; and more than 10 METs during cross-country skiing.

As you progress in your tolerance for exercise and build up your strength through conditioning, you and your doctor will use the term MET when talking about what you should and should not be doing. As you will see, all activities are classified according to the number of METs required to perform them. Some of the lower MET activities you may be able to do right now; others you can look forward to doing in the near future.

The MET system is an extremely useful shorthand for establishing and carrying out a progressive approach to recovery. You begin by performing one group of activities at a certain MET level. When your doctor believes that you can do these safely and your body is able to do more, you move up to the next MET level of activities. Eventually, you should attain that level of fitness you and your doctor feel is best for your optimal level of good health. (Don't expect to work up to the 10 METs or more level. Chances are your doctor will suggest that you stop before you reach that point.)

Here's a list of the MET levels of a few simple activities:

1 MET

Sleeping
Sitting in a chair
Lying in bed

2 METs

Standing
Walking 1 mph
Reading
Writing a letter
Working at a desk
Playing cards and table games
Sedentary hobbies performed at a table
Hand sewing
Light dusting
Typing (electric)
Shaving
Dressing
Brushing your hair

2–3 METs

Entertaining a few visitors
Typing (manual)
Washing your hair
Peeling vegetables
Folding laundry
Walking at 2 mph
Horseback riding (walking pace)
Bowling
Playing the piano
Playing golf (motorized cart)

3–4 METs

Doing the laundry (light loads)
Ironing
Washing by hand
Making the bed
Flying (if doctor permits)
Meal preparations
Driving a car in an uncongested area
Walking at 3 mph
Going out to dinner, the movies, concerts, etc.
Pulling a cart
Cleaning windows
Handling a small boat
Driving a truck
Climbing stairs (slowly)
Bicycling at 6 mph
Playing golf (pulling a cart)

4–5 METs

Mopping floors
Driving in heavy traffic
Playing badminton
Walking at 4 mph
Taking out the garbage (using a dolly)

Light gardening
Ballroom dancing (not rock and roll)
Painting or hanging wallpaper
Attending meetings
Raking leaves
Light carpentry

5–6 METs

Bicycling at 8 mph
Fishing in a stream
Tennis (doubles)
Rollerskating
Light shoveling and digging

6–7 METs

Tennis (singles)
Walking at 5 mph
Light downhill skiing
Waterskiing
Square dancing
Splitting wood
Shoveling snow
Lawn mowing

7–8 METs

Jogging at 5 mph
Bicycling at 12 mph
Downhill skiing
Horseback riding (canter to gallop)
Canoeing
Playing football

8–9 METs

Running at 5½ mph
Bicycling at 13 mph
Cross-country skiing
Playing basketball

10 OR MORE METs

Playing handball or squash
Climbing a slope with a heavy load
Running at 6 mph
Running at 8 mph (13½ METs)
Running at 13 mph (17 METs)

Look at all the activities in your MET level. If you are able to walk 3 miles per hour (a 3–4 MET activity), you should be able to bicycle at 6 miles per hour or go out to dinner with a few friends. The above list is just a general description, however; the exact MET expenditure associated with a particular exercise depends on several variables—your skill, how often you pause to rest, weather conditions and, of course, the state of your health. Before you try any new activity, check not just with the MET list but with your doctor as well.

TAKING YOUR PULSE

In order to use the MET system as efficiently as possible, you have to learn how to measure your heart rate, or pulse. Just press the index and middle fingers of one hand on the wrist of the other, palm side up, and count the number of beats you feel for a period of 10 seconds. It helps to have a partner watch the clock while you count. Then multiply the number of beats by six. This will tell you how many times your heart is beating per minute. Some people find that the pulse on the wrist isn't quite strong enough. If you're one of them, try pressing your fingertips lightly but firmly on the side of your neck just under the jawbone.

It's important to take your pulse whenever trying a new activity, even if your doctor has given you the go-ahead. It's best to take the measurement while still in motion, but if that is not possible, be sure to do it immediately after stopping or the reading you get will not be accurate. Your heart rate slows down very quickly even after a short delay.

There are several devices on the market that actually measure your pulse for you by giving you a digital readout whenever you need it. They're certainly not necessary—and they are expensive—but check them out if you wish.

YOUR TARGET HEART RATE

Now that you know how to take your pulse, it's time to learn what the information you've gained is good for. That's where your target heart rate comes into play. Your target heart rate is the number of beats per minute at which you can safely exercise while still improving the physical condition of your body. If your heart rate is too high, you may be endangering your health; if it's too low, you're not working hard enough.

Your target heart rate helps you to strike a balance between being overly cautious and overly energetic. If you sit in a chair and just move your arms, it's probably safe to say that you're not overexerting yourself. In fact, the activity probably increases your heart rate by a scant five beats per minute. At the other extreme, if you leap out of your chair and start jumping rope, your heart might beat as many as 100 extra beats per minute. You might be conditioning your body, but you might also be straining yourself beyond your limits. And that's what the target heart rate is all about—setting limits.

The best way to establish a target heart rate is to undergo an exercise stress test on a treadmill. Your doctor will usually do this at the start of your conditioning phase, and it's also a routine part of every cardiac rehabilitation program.

One rough way to calculate your target heart rate is by means of simple math. Subtract your age from 220 and then multiply that number by .60. For example, if you're fifty years old, you subtract 50 from 220 and get 170. Then you multiply 170 by .60 and get a target heart rate of 102 beats per minute. If you're taking beta blocker medication, which slows down your heart rate, you'll figure your heart rate a little differently: Subtract your age from 220, multiply the result by .60, and then subtract 20. If the fifty-year-old patient described above was taking beta blockers, the target heart rate would be 82.

However you compute your target heart rate, be sure that you check your figures with your doctor or the staff at the cardiac rehabilitation center before you engage in any exercise. Knowing your target heart rate is an invaluable method of determining how fast you should be exercising, but the number is helpful only if it's accurate.

Suppose you are about to embark on a half-hour walk, and you want to know how fast your pace should be. You start walking for five minutes at a slow speed and then, still walking, check your pulse. If your target heart rate is 112 and your pulse rate is only 100, you know you aren't walking fast enough. Pick up the pace for five minutes and take another reading. If you're up around 125, slow down a little until you can get your heart rate to between 110 and 115 beats per minute.

You can use your target heart rate as a guide for all your daily activities. Consider the fifty-year-old patient with a target rate of 102. Fifteen minutes into the walk he or she checks his or her pulse and finds that it's between 100 and 105 beats per minute, exactly where it should be. At this point the speed of the walk should be calculated as closely as possible. If, for example, it took 30 minutes to walk a mile, that's 2 miles per hour. Looking at the list of METs activities in this chapter, we find that our patient has performed a 2–3 MET task. As long as a doctor approves, he or she should be able to do all the other things in the 2–3 MET level.

Eventually you will find that the energy required to perform the activities in a given MET level won't be enough to attain your target heart rate. After about 10 days of walking at a very slow pace, many patients find that their measured heart rates are 10 to 15 beats slower than their target heart rates. This drop is a good sign; it means that increased physical conditioning has helped your heart, your circulatory system, and your leg muscles to operate more efficiently. It also means that your body is ready for more challenges.

At this point, after clearing it with your doctor, you should increase your walking speed to 2½ or 3 miles per hour, which should bring your heart rate back up to the target zone of 102 beats per minute. Since walking at 3 miles per hour without fatigue is a 3–4 MET activity, you should be able to do other things listed at this level.

After you've been involved in the conditioning program for about six weeks, your doctor will probably teach you some new math, asking you to compute your heart rate a little differently. You'll still subtract your age from 220, but you'll now multiply that figure by .65 instead of .60. This will change not only your target heart rate but also the amount of exercise you'll be doing in a half-hour of conditioning.

Think of your target rate as a helpful tool you and your doctor can use during your recovery. Also, consider it with a certain amount of pride. Increasing your target rate means you are getting closer and closer to optimum physical health, closer and closer to reaching your goals.

HOW TO EXERCISE

The most important aspect of your exercise program during the conditioning phase (or any phase, for that matter) can be summed up in one word: *safety*. When you are engaged in physical exertion, always keep in mind that you have limitations. And remember too that you should be exercising only with the approval of a doctor who is aware of the state of your health and your conditioning routine.

Even if you feel as if you can take on the world, do everything in moderation. Do your warm-up and cool-down exercises faithfully and at a leisurely pace. There are no hard and fast rules about the minimum exercise time, but generally your workout shouldn't last longer than about 30 minutes, not including warm-up and cool-down time. Build slowly to your highest level of physical exertion. If you are walking, take the first 5 minutes at a leisurely pace. After that, start walking briskly in order to reach and maintain your target heart rate. Then, 25 minutes after you begin, start to slow down again, resuming your leisurely pace for the last 5 minutes.

Finally, alert your doctor immediately the moment any of the following occurs:

- Heavy pressure or squeezing pain in the chest that spreads to the shoulder, arms, neck, or jaw and is not relieved by rest and/or nitroglycerin tablets within 10 minutes
- Increased shortness of breath or coughing
- Overall weakness
- Swelling of the feet or ankles, especially in the morning
- Fainting or dizziness
- Slow or rapid heart rate (usually below 50 or above 140 beats per minute)
- Irregular heartbeat

HOW OFTEN TO EXERCISE

In the conditioning phase you should try to exercise every day, but if that's not possible, you should get in 30 minutes at least three times a week. The more often you exercise, the more quickly you will get your body into shape. Don't go more than three or four days in a row without exercising. Doctors have found that after just 10 days of inactivity, patients begin to lose the effects of their conditioning, and after just one month without exercise, nearly all of their efforts are lost.

If you do stop for a month or more, you'll have to start conditioning again at a low MET level, gradually building up to the level of physical fitness you had before you stopped exercising. You will have to recalculate your target heart rates, returning to the multiplication factor of .60 for about six weeks. After six weeks of renewed regular conditioning, most patients can return to the .65 factor.

Of course, if you're not well enough to exercise, you have no choice but to stop temporarily. If you should get sick and find you simply cannot engage in strenuous physical activities, you should follow your doctor's recommendations for rest and recovery. Once you recuperate, you will be able to resume your exercise program at a lower MET rate.

BEATING THE HEAT

It's best to exercise when the temperature is above 55°F (13°C) and below 80°F (27°C). If the weather is particularly hot, humid, or cold, consider exercising inside—walking around in an enclosed shopping mall, supermarket, or hotel/motel complex, for example, or enrolling in a nearby health club. In the summer get in the habit of taking a walk early in the morning.

No matter how hot or humid it is, and no matter how much you'd like to rush into a refreshing shower immediately after exercising, don't. Wait at least an hour after exercising to take your shower, and then use only lukewarm water. A postexercise shower must never be very hot or very cold.

CHOOSING THE RIGHT EXERCISE

Perhaps the best way to stick to your exercise program is to make it as convenient and as enjoyable as possible, and that means, among other things, that it doesn't require a lot of equipment or perfect weather. If you led a sedentary life before your heart attack—and it's very likely that you did—you can now explore which sports suit you best. For example, if you don't like walking and can't imagine using a stationary bicycle, ask your doctor about other options, such as swimming, nonimpact aerobics, or other activities that will heighten your endurance. Have a couple of activities to fall back on in case of inclement weather or out-of-town travel. As long as the activity is approved by your doctor, choose a form of exercise that makes you happy.

Warm-up and Cool-down Exercises

During the conditioning phase, you should continue to take the time for some brief warm-up and cool-down routines every time you exercise. However, you will find that the warm-ups and cool-downs during the conditioning phase are much more vigorous than those in the convalescent phase.

It's important not to rush your warm-ups and cool-downs. Since the whole idea of these exercises is to prepare for increased (or decreased) activity, you should not shock your body with overexertion. It is best if you concentrate on doing them at a leisurely, comfortable pace.

The exercises are illustrated and described on this and the following pages. Make a copy of them and keep it handy.

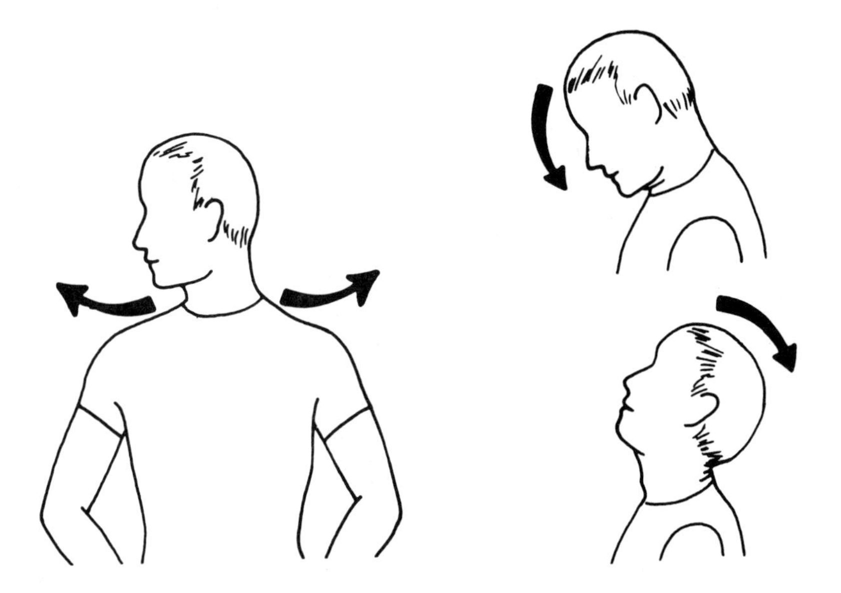

Head Rotation. Stand up straight with your hands on your hips and your feet spread shoulder width apart. Slowly turn your head from side to side and from front to back. Repeat three times.

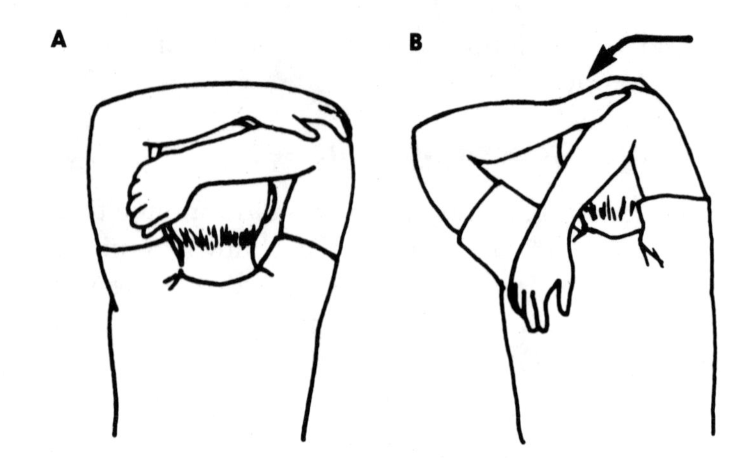

Shoulder Stretch 1. Hold your elbow with the opposite hand (A) and gently pull it back behind your head (B). This will stretch your shoulder and the back of your arms. Hold the stretch gently for 30 seconds. It is not important how far you can stretch; it is important how good the stretch feels to you. Repeat the exercise once, using the other elbow and hand.

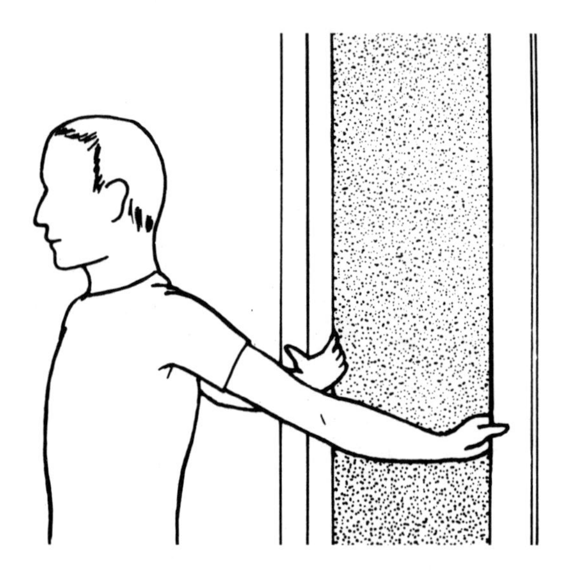

Shoulder Stretch 2. With your back to a fence or a doorway and your arms at shoulder level, reach backward and grab either the top of the fence or the sides of the doorway. Lean forward, keeping your chest and head up and straightening your arms. Hold this stretch for 20 seconds. Do this exercise only once.

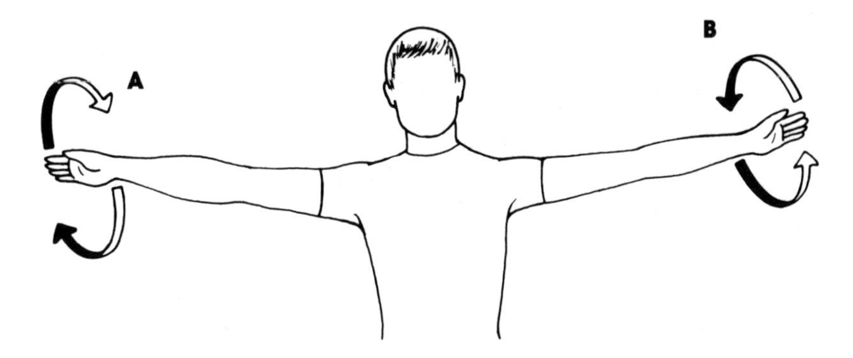

Arm Circulation. Stand up straight, legs slightly apart. Extend your arms out to either side and start to move them forward in small circles (A). Gradually make the circles bigger, stopping when they are as big as you can make them. Reverse the direction, moving your arms backward in circles (B). Repeat five times.

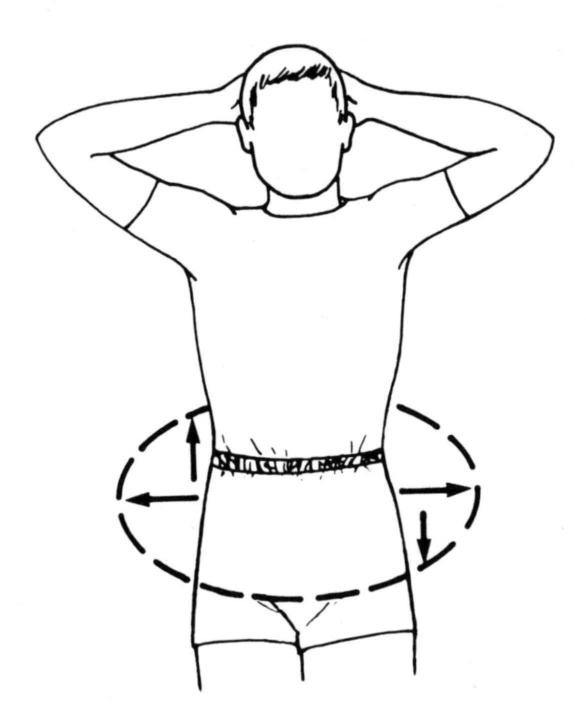

Trunk Rotation. Stand up straight, with your feet shoulder width apart. Put your hands behind your head and rotate your trunk to the right, back, left, and front. Reverse the direction and repeat. Do this exercise only once in each direction.

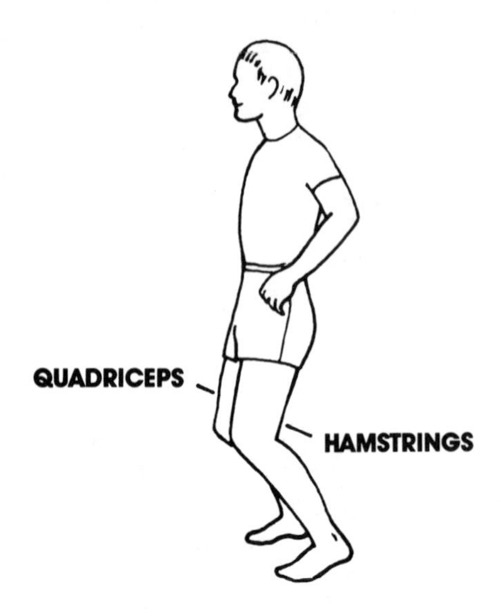

Quarter-squat. Stand up straight, with your legs slightly apart. Lower yourself into a quarter-squat position and hold this position for 30 seconds. This relaxes your hamstrings and makes it easier to stretch during exercise.

Walking

Walking is probably the safest and simplest activity during your conditioning phase. It requires no special equipment, it can be done anywhere at virtually any time, and if you choose a scenic spot, it can be a feast for the eyes as well as the heart. It can even be sociable, since many people are discovering the joys of walking for health. If you feel like having company on your daily walk, you probably won't have to look far.

Jogging

Some patients may progress from walking to jogging, but the progression is by no means automatic. Even slow jogging is a 7–8 MET activity, and getting strong enough for that takes time. You should never jog unless your doctor specifically approves the sport. Jogging immediately after a heart attack can be potentially dangerous, even fatal. Only through slow, progressive physical conditioning can you make jogging a reasonable form of activity.

Stationary Bicycles

In general, outdoor bicycling is not recommended in the conditioning phase; it requires vigorous activity, and it introduces the additional threat of traffic. If you want a change from walking, consider renting, borrowing, or buying a stationary bicycle. You can adjust the controls of a stationary bike so that you get the workout you need, and you can do it all in the safety of your living room.

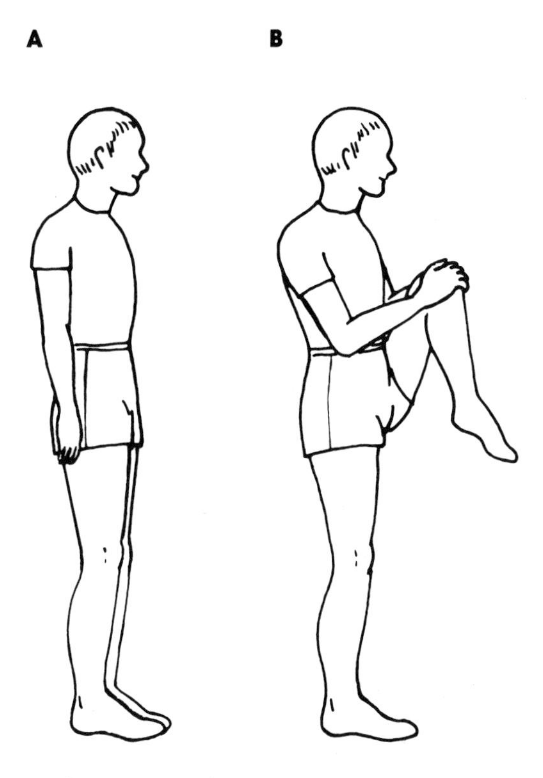

Knee Presses. Stand up straight, hands at your sides (A). Lift your right knee to your chest (B) and press it close to your chest with your hand. Exhale. Repeat exercise with left leg. Do this exercise twice for each leg.

Be sure to use your target heart rate to assess your progress on the bicycle, just as you would if you were walking. And don't forget to do your warm-ups and cool-downs. If you find "riding nowhere" boring, putting the bike in front of the television or listening to the radio during your workouts may help to pass the time.

Treadmills

Since treadmills play such an important part in the testing you undergo in cardiac rehabilitation, and since the idea of being

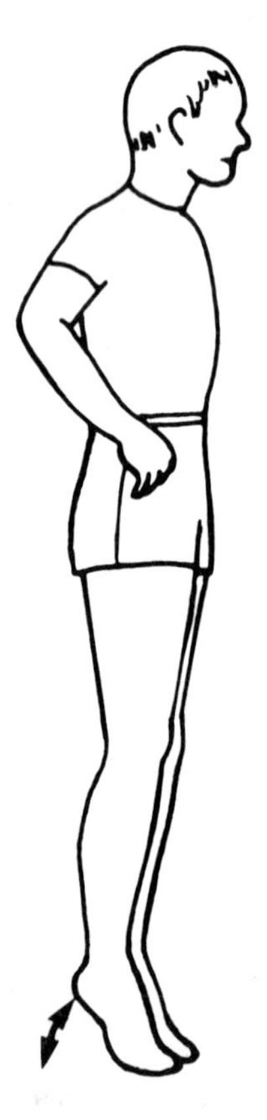

Toe Raises. Standing with your feet 6 inches apart, put your hands on your hips and push up and down on your toes. Repeat 15 times.

able to walk at a steady pace in all kinds of weather is so appealing, at some time along the way you may consider using a treadmill for your regular daily exercise. Many health clubs now have treadmills in the equipment room, and if you know how to use one and you have the approval of your doctor, you can feel free to do so.

If you are thinking about buying a treadmill, ask your doctor about the best kind to choose. He or she will probably tell you that the only ones worth having are the heavy-duty medical treadmills. Naturally, they're the most expensive ones.

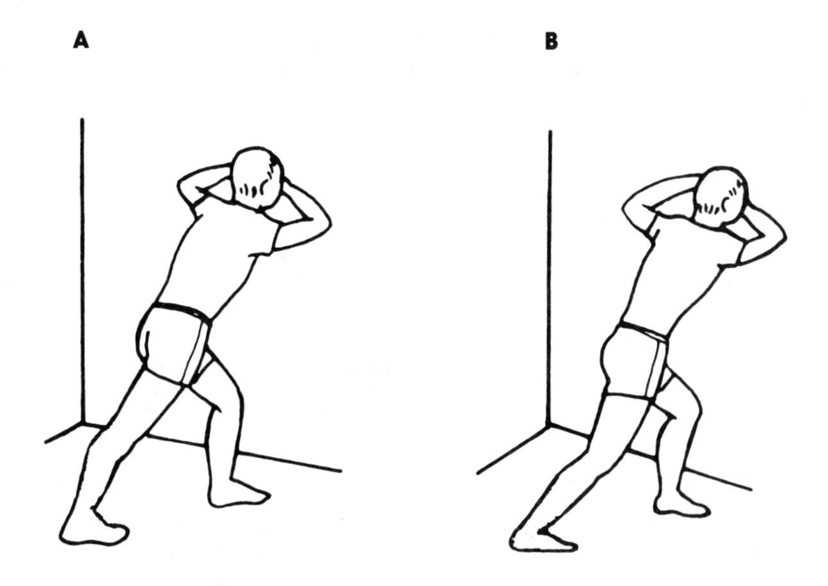

Leg Stretch A. Standing a little away from a wall, lean on it with your forearms and rest your head on your hands. Bend one knee and place your foot forward, leaving the other leg straight out behind you. Move your hips forward until you feel the stretch in the calf of your straight leg. Keep both heels on the ground and toes straight ahead. Hold for 30 seconds. (Do not rock back and forth or bounce.) Repeat with other leg. **Leg Stretch B.** Follow instructions for leg stretch A, but this time bend your back knee slightly, keeping your foot flat. (You will get a much lower stretch and maintain good ankle flexibility when doing this.) Hold the stretch for 15 seconds and repeat with the other leg.

Sports

As you may have guessed, this is not the time to go out for pro football or train for the Boston Marathon. Yes, it's true that during the conditioning phase you should start a conscientious exercise program, but it's also true that you must be very careful about which activities you choose.

Competitive sports are a mixed bag. On the one hand, they're usually fun, and you'll probably be inclined to stick to a schedule of activities you really enjoy. On the other hand, they may be too vigorous; you may get so caught up in the heat of the game that you forget that what you're there for is safe, sensible conditioning. You also may lose track of the time and forget to stop to measure your heart rate. In time you may be able to enjoy a carefree set of doubles or some other competitive sport, but for now it's probably best to avoid even friendly competition.

Sit down with your doctor and go over your options. Some of the sports your doctor may suggest are table tennis, golf, calisthenics, and cycling, all of which require smooth, continuous action and give your heart and circulatory system a consistent, steady workout. Swimming is good, too, as long as the water is neither too hot nor too cold. Check with your doctor about the style of your stroke and the distance you plan to swim during your exercise sessions.

Be wary of activities that involve short, intermittent bursts of energy. No matter how much you enjoy them, tennis, squash, and handball aren't appropriate activities for the conditioning phase of your recovery. Neither are isometric exercises—water skiing, downhill skiing, pushups, and situps, for example—which concentrate energy in only a few areas of the body.

Always be aware that there are limits to what you can do. It may not be a particularly pleasant thought, but it could save your life.

TRAVELING

Yes, you most definitely may pack your bags and travel during your conditioning phase. You are not to think of yourself as an invalid. However, if you do plan to get away for a while, keep the following advice in mind:

- If you're traveling by car, stop every hour. Get out of the car and walk around for a few minutes to revive your circulation.
- Make sure you have your doctor's approval before you travel by plane. Once you're in the air, it's a good idea to get up every hour or so and take a walk up and down the aisles.
- Make sure you have your doctor's approval before you go to a place with an extremely warm or extremely cold climate or somewhere with an altitude above 6,000 feet. You will probably be allowed to go on the trip, but you'll have to take special precautions.
- Remember to take an adequate supply of your medication. I always suggest that patients take enough for an extra week in case they decide to stay longer.
- Carry a summary of your medical history with you and, if possible, a recent EKG.
- When you reach your destination, make sure you know where the nearest hospital, emergency department, and physician can be located. Do not dwell upon the possibility of an emergency, but be prepared if trouble should occur.

SAYING "NO"

In some ways one of the hardest aspects of the conditioning phase is reminding yourself not to do too much. You may be feeling wonderful and looking so fit that your friends and business associates have completely forgotten about the heart attack you had a few months ago. Without thinking they may ask you to do more than you're ready for. Remember your limitations. As difficult as it may seem sometimes, you have to learn to say "no."

RETURNING TO WORK

About six to eight weeks after your heart attack, your doctor will probably give you the green light to return to work. This is not an okay to charge into the office and resume your old, stressful patterns. Take it slowly; gradually ease yourself back into the job.

It can be helpful to simulate work activity at home before you actually return to the office. If you have a desk job, sit at a desk at home for a couple of hours and try to figure out typical work problems. (Think back to some of the decisions you made on the job and rework them with a slightly different scenario.) If you have a manufacturing or labor-intensive occupation, do something that approximates what you do at work. Be careful not to exert yourself too much. Talk to your doctor about how you'll be getting to work. If you normally drive on congested freeways, consider joining a car pool instead or take public transportation to and from the office.

Once you're back on the job, you should expect things to be somewhat different. At first, your co-workers may seem extremely inquisitive, wanting to know all that happened to you. Understand that part of their interest may be due to their need for reassurance—not just that it isn't going to happen to you again but that it isn't going to happen to them. And then there are the people who are just insatiably curious about things medical; they'll want a blow-by-blow description of your entire ordeal. Do whatever seems comfortable for you. If you feel like talking about it, go ahead. If you'd rather not discuss it, say so, politely but firmly.

If your regular job involves physical labor, you may have discovered that you've been assigned less strenuous tasks than usual when you first get back. Do not interpret this change as a demotion; a transfer out of a situation in which you were at risk of another heart attack is for your own good. Of course, it's for the company's good as well. If you have a second heart attack because of your work environment, your employer may risk having to pay hefty workers' compensation costs.

You are also responsible for making some changes on your own. Now that you know the dangers of stress, do your best to stay away from stressful situations. Avoid unnecessary arguments; learn to delegate some responsibilities; take relaxation breaks. If your work situation remains as stressful as it was before your heart attack, consider changing jobs for the sake of your physical and mental well-being.

Changing Jobs

Many people have used their heart attacks as an impetus for switching jobs. For them, a brush with death made them realize the importance of living life to its fullest.

One of my patients got involved in a new career almost by accident. He'd been a successful accountant for 15 years, but April 15 finally caught up with him, and he had a fairly serious heart attack. While he was home convalescing, he got bored with reading and watching television, so he decided to putter around in the kitchen. He had virtually never boiled an egg before this time, but he discovered a real flair for cooking. When his doctor gave him permission, he took a few cooking classes, and after that he never looked back. Today he runs a thriving catering business, and to remind himself of the old days, he always takes a vacation during the first two weeks of April.

If you feel that a change is in order for you, bear in mind that the key to switching jobs is to make sure, as much as you can, that you're making a change for the better, one that will give you more pleasure and cause less stress in your life than the one you have. Do not make a transition that may cause you financial setbacks. And remember, change itself may cause stress. If you are unsure of the consequences of your actions, you might do well to postpone making a dramatic change. This is not a good time to gamble.

Whatever you decide to do—go back to your old job or make a change—it makes sense to consult a psychologist first. A professional can offer advice on starting afresh or returning to your former employer and help you set realistic goals. Vocational guidance may also be of some help.

15

The Psychology of Healing

Two of my patients underwent heart surgery at about the same time. One was forty-five years old, and the other was fifty-two. Their risk factors were very similar: both were smokers; both had hypertension, elevated stress levels, and high cholesterol counts; both were about 20 pounds overweight. But there was one major difference between them—their psychological outlooks.

The forty-five-year-old faced recovery with a positive outlook. He quit smoking right away, ate a modified diet, was diligent about taking periodic relaxation breaks, and didn't hesitate to enroll in a cardiac rehabilitation program. Total recovery was his ultimate goal, and he promised his family and friends that he was going to make it.

The behavior of the fifty-two-year-old was precisely the opposite. He said he couldn't give up smoking, and he continued to eat the high-fat foods he was used to. He attended cardiac rehabilitation classes but only because "the doctor said I had to go." As far as this patient was concerned, recovery was horrible, and life after a heart attack was nothing but deprivation and the constant fear of the unknown.

Which patient recovered faster? You can probably guess. Within several weeks the patient with the positive outlook was off his blood pressure medication, and his cholesterol level had plummeted. Just as he had vowed, it appeared that full recovery was all but certain. My other patient was still on his medication, and his cholesterol level was still elevated. Six months after cardiac rehabilitation, the prognosis for his full recovery was still questionable.

The moral of this story is, quite simply, that when it comes to cardiac rehabilitation, or practically anything else for that matter, your psychological outlook is critically important. How you think and feel about your future has a lot to do not just with how fast you'll recover but also with whether you'll recover at all.

I can hear you saying, "Sure, it's all very well to say that I should think positive. But how do I do it?" I hope that the rest of this chapter will help you answer that question, by dealing with the common psychological concerns of many patients and some effective ways of overcoming them.

If you're serious about trying to improve your psychological outlook, the first thing you have to do is to tell yourself that you owe yourself the best recovery possible. This means a bright outlook about the future as well as coming to terms with the past. Consider the following information and then have your doctor help you tailor it to suit your own needs. You have to be comfortable with a psychological program if it is going to help you. Everyone has different needs, attitudes, and social support networks that help us cope with a crisis. What works for one person may not work for another.

CONQUERING DEPRESSION

No matter how determined you are to be upbeat in your outlook, don't expect every day to be an "up" day after your heart attack. In fact, depression following a heart attack is quite common. Most patients complain of feeling powerless and apprehensive about the future, at least once in a while. If you are young, you may be feeling resentful too, because you think you've been robbed of your best years. If you are more than sixty, you may begin to think that you are entering the final stages of life. Neither of these feelings is true, but both are common, and both are understandable. Normally they pass quite quickly.

There are ways to speed things up, too. Exercise can be an excellent method of conquering depression. It takes your mind off your concerns, and at the same time it bolsters your self-esteem and enhances your sense of independence. Remember the feeling you had when you took your first walk around the block after the heart attack? Chances are you felt proud that you had the stamina to do it alone, without the help of a doctor, nurse, or relative. Exercise is almost always a foolproof means of fighting depression.

Another way you can ward off depression and fear is by learning more about your condition. Once you know what happened to you during the heart attack and what is going on during recovery, you'll be more rational in determining your future. Sit down with your doctors and nurses and ask questions. Keep a list of questions as they occur to you. Show the professionals that you're interested in knowing about your illness. Tell them that you want to take an active part in your recovery.

Reading can help, too. This book is a good start, but there are other resources to which you can turn. Have a look at the list of books and pamphlets listed at the back of this book and send away for literature from the American Heart Association. Contact the national office of the AHA at 7320 Greenville Avenue, Dallas, Texas 75221, or try a local chapter in the city nearest you.

Exercise and education are helpful if you're feeling a little down, but they're not always the answer. If you are suffering from extremely severe depression, you should alert your physician. Here are some warning signs that may indicate that your depression is worthy of concern:

- Weight loss that is not attributable to dieting
- Difficulty in getting to sleep and/or remaining asleep (this usually means waking up early in the morning and not being able to get back to sleep again)
- Constipation not attributable to eating habits
- Lack of interest in sex
- Preoccupation with death or suicide
- Lack of interest in your family and friends
- Loss of interest in hobbies or any other activity you used to enjoy
- Worrying excessively about trivialities
- Difficulty in concentrating
- Carelessness about your clothes and personal appearance

Severe depression can be a serious impediment to your recovery. If you notice the symptoms of depression, see your physician immediately. The sooner you can get back on track, the sooner you can get on with your recovery.

DENIAL

"I didn't have a heart attack. Those were only chest pains from something I ate."

"I didn't have a heart attack. A friend of mine said that those enzyme tests don't mean anything."

"I didn't have a heart attack. I don't smoke, and I hardly ever eat red meat."

I can't tell you how many times I've heard patients make those or similar remarks. If you've ever heard yourself say any of them, it's time for you to think long and hard about your health. You may have a serious problem with denial.

Denial is remarkably widespread among heart attack patients. In one significant heart attack study in which I participated, 345 men were interviewed three weeks after they had been hospitalized for a heart attack. Of these, 20 percent denied that they had heart problems at all. What's more, most of these "deniers" refused to heed their doctors' advice. Many continued to smoke and overeat; others blatantly overexerted themselves.

Denial is a natural reaction—after all, none of us likes to accept bad news—but if it's allowed to continue, it can be a serious, even deadly problem. Your refusal to admit you had a heart attack may lead you to refuse proper treatment. Even worse, you could refuse to admit you're having a second heart attack and ignore the fact that you need immediate, life-saving assistance.

Why do so many people deny they've had heart attacks? Psychologists believe that denial is a coping mechanism. By denying that they had a heart attack, heart patients can protect themselves from the worry, fear, and (yes) responsibilities of a heart attack victim. When I have a patient with a denial problem, here are some of the suggestions I make:

- **Educate yourself.** The enemy you know is better than the enemy you don't know.

- **Join a cardiac rehabilitation group.** The group support will help you to acknowledge your vulnerability and encourage you to comply with the advice of your physician.
- **Participate in a physical therapy program.** Physical therapy is usually included in a cardiac rehabilitation program, but if you're not enrolled in a structured rehabilitation course, you should still ask your doctor to recommend a licensed physical therapist. The therapist will help you come to grips with the state of your health, but even more important, he or she will help you set and achieve realistic fitness goals without overexercising your healing heart.

PROJECTION

Like denial, projection, which is characterized by blaming other people or incidents for your health setbacks, is a typical reaction of heart attack patients. For example, you may blame your spouse or family for your heart attack because there was tension between you before the incident. "If I hadn't had to pick up your dirty clothes, I never would have had the heart attack!" and "If you hadn't been kicked out of school, I wouldn't be in the hospital today!" are just two of the heated accusations I've heard in the last few months. Or you might blame your parents for passing on a family history of heart disease.

Again, this kind of reaction is understandable, and under normal circumstances a patient will soon realize that blaming others is irrational, not to mention counterproductive. If the projection continues, you should probably talk to a psychologist about your feelings. Projection can harm your relationship with your loved ones and seriously hinder your recovery. Instead of blaming others for the heart attack you just had, focus on the present and the future.

OBSESSIVE COMPULSION

One patient of mine spent hours formulating an elaborate plan for every step in the convalescent phase of her recovery. She prepared elaborate meal plans, complete with calorie, fat, and cholesterol counts, and insisted that her husband hire a full-time cook. She became an exercise fanatic, boring her friends and family with stories about her target heart rate. She made her daily walk into a drawn-out, overblown ritual. And she became hypercritical of others, yelling at anyone who ate rich foods in front of her or smoked a cigarette anywhere within breathing range. In short, after her heart attack, my patient became an obsessive compulsive.

Obsessive compulsion is characterized by extreme fastidiousness and attention to detail in the steps you make toward recovery. The best way to overcome obsessive compulsion is to recognize your extreme behavior and confront it. Following a routine can be useful during recovery, but if you make your daily affairs unusually long and drawn out, force yourself to break free from the ritual you created. Changing your routine will not kill you; it may help you to progress.

THE NAGGING PROBLEM

I'll never forget the expression on the face of one of my patients when he said (or should I say shrieked?): "If another heart attack doesn't kill me, the nagging from my friends and family will!"

I can't say that I blamed him for feeling so frustrated. He had been having a rough time sticking to his diet and exercise program, and his family had been coming down on him pretty hard. He felt bad enough about backsliding without being nagged about it. I gave him the best advice I could think of: be patient. I reminded him that his loved ones were smothering him with their concern because they wanted to help. If they could diet and exercise for him, they would, I said, but since they can't, they remind him to diet and exercise. Nagging is their way of demonstrating how much they care.

Then I had a talk with his wife and children. I sympathized with them too, but I explained to them how their well-intentioned nagging was making my patient feel. I told them that a relationship may suffer when someone you love constantly reminds you what is best for you. What's more, the situation may interfere with a patient's recovery.

Nagging is an emotional response you and your loved ones must overcome together. How to solve the nagging problem? Here are a few tips that should help:

1. Be honest with yourself. Are you overeating, not exercising, or ignoring your doctor's orders? Are you unconsciously asking your family to function as supervisors? Are you forcing them to nag you? Talk this possibility over with your family.
2. If you are convinced that you're doing everything possible to help in your recovery, say so. Explain to your family why you feel their nagging is unjustified.
3. Encourage those close to you to join you in learning about heart attack recovery. If you all learn about the healing process together, you are less likely to be smothered by misguided concern.
4. Recognize that nagging may be caused by acute emotional overload. Perhaps the nagger is upset by a number of problems and merely using you as an emotional outlet. Try to discuss this possibility with the nagger, but be as tactful and as understanding as possible. You're the patient, but everyone involved with your heart attack has suffered.
5. If you are in a cardiac rehabilitation program, inquire about group psychotherapy programs for families. Many

rehabilitation facilities offer such programs for a small fee or even free of charge. The sessions usually are informal, and they often provide much welcome relief.

If none of the above suggestions works, describe the situation to your doctor. He may have some suggestions or recommend additional professional help. Above all, keep in mind that understanding each other's reactions, fears, and needs is of the utmost importance right now. This is no time for family fights. A "house divided" cannot recover from a heart attack.

MEDICATION

There are many medications that can help you through the psychological problems you may encounter during your recovery. For example, your doctor may prescribe a sedative to calm you down or may suggest that you take a nonprescription tension-reliever, such as a sleeping aid. Most of these contain a small dose of antihistamine, which produces a sedative effect.

Remember that any and all medications you take must be prescribed or approved by your doctor and must be taken precisely as prescribed. Never take anyone else's medication, no matter how harmless it appears to be. And keep in mind that while certain drugs may be safe by themselves, they can be deadly when mixed with alcohol.

PROFESSIONAL ASSISTANCE

If the suggestions made throughout this chapter have not improved your psychological outlook, you may need to see a professional counselor or psychotherapist. If you do decide to seek professional help, don't regard this as a sign of weakness or failure. The fact is, it is one of the smartest and bravest things you can do to help yourself.

If your body is in pain, you see a medical doctor. If your emotions are causing you pain, you should consult a mental health professional. Many people who don't understand psychology or psychiatry call the doctors who specialize in these fields "shrinks," but they couldn't be more wrong. A better name for these people would be "expanders," because of the valuable work they do in making people expand their awareness.

How do you find the right professional help? Your doctor can describe the many kinds of psychological assistance available to you and provide you with a reliable referral. Here are the basic choices your doctor will describe:

- **Psychiatrist.** In terms of training, the psychiatrist has the most extensive background. A psychiatrist is a physician, schooled in the functioning of the body and licensed to prescribe medications. If you have a physical problem that affects your emotional situation (or vice versa), a psychiatrist can provide the help you need.
- **Psychologist.** A psychologist deals more with personality theory and psychological testing than with the functioning of the body. A psychologist probably will give you an extensive personality evaluation to help you understand your emotions. Some psychologists are brilliant psychotherapists, but a psychologist is not a physician and may not prescribe medications.
- **Psychotherapist.** Another direction you may consider is psychotherapy, which is usually conducted by a mental health counselor. You may choose individual or group psychotherapy, depending on which makes you feel more comfortable. You may even consider family psychotherapy, since your loved ones are so intimately

involved in your recovery. Typically, psychotherapy helps you gain insights into your emotions and coping mechanisms. It also helps you identify and modify behavior that may be interfering with your recovery. The mental health counselor may not prescribe medications.

16 Money Matters

When you're recovering from a heart attack, the last thing that should be on your mind is your checkbook. Unfortunately, that's not the way it usually is. Most patients begin to worry about finances soon after coming home from the hospital. That's perfectly understandable, since that's when the medical bills start coming in. Health care costs are high, and when you begin to tally the total when they're added to the regular household bills, you may begin to feel that you're headed for the poorhouse. As you sit down and try to balance your checkbook, your state of mind is not likely to be conducive to rehabilitation.

Your first step? Hand over that checkbook! Give it to your spouse, one of your children, your accountant—anyone you can trust. Even if you think you can manage money at this time, you shouldn't try. You have enough on your mind already.

Letting go of the family purse strings is very difficult for some people, but at least one patient I know, a fifty-seven-year-old businessman who was hospitalized after a very serious heart attack, reaped unexpected benefits when he turned the family's financial responsibilities over to his wife. His wife hadn't paid the bills in thirty years; in fact, her ineptitude with money had become something of a joke in the family. But since my patient was going to have to be in the hospital for at least six weeks, he didn't have much choice but to let someone else handle the checkbook for a while. I persuaded him to let his wife have a go at it.

Eight weeks later, when he went home from the hospital, my patient took a tentative look at the checkbook and was delighted to discover that everything was in perfect order. Promising never to joke about her lack of financial acumen again, he handed the checkbook back to her—for good. A few months after my patient left the hospital his wife told me somewhat sheepishly, that she had always felt a little like a second-class citizen when it came to money. Being able to step in and take over an important role in managing the family did wonders for her self-esteem, and their marriage.

So take my advice: turn your checkbook over to a caretaker, at least temporarily. And after you've read through the rest of this chapter, ask him or her to read it too.

FINANCING CARDIAC REHABILITATION

Most private insurance plans will pay for at least part of your cardiac rehabilitation after you leave the hospital, but be sure to read the fine print on the policy. Some cover only 80 percent of the program's costs and put restrictions on the number of weeks you may participate. Medicare usually pays for 12 weeks of cardiac rehabilitation (three sessions a week), but Medicaid (the program for needy individuals of any age) doesn't cover cardiac rehabilitation programs at all in most states.

The number of sessions and the cost of cardiac rehabilitation programs vary throughout the country. At the moment there are no exact rules that govern what a program must offer.

Some cardiac rehabilitation programs feature carefully monitored exercise sessions; others have no patient monitoring. After you've discussed various cardiac rehabilitation programs with your doctor, check with your insurance company about the terms for reimbursement. Before you make a decision, visit the business office of the rehabilitation program you are considering. Most programs offer financial advice to potential participants.

FAMILY FINANCES

Even if your health insurance situation is relatively secure, you may still have money worries. After all, insurance plans don't pay the electric bill! Besides, you may be feeling apprehensive about losing time from work.

If money is tight, be assured that there are ways to manage your bills after a heart attack. You or the person tending your checkbook should arrange your bills in the order of importance. See what the penalty is for late payment and whether or not the creditor will disrupt your service if you put off paying for a little longer. For example, department stores will usually wait longer for your check than the telephone company will.

With nearly all creditors you can make special arrangements for partial payments. In many instances, writing a small check is better than paying nothing at all. Have your spouse or financial counselor call each biller to ask if you can establish a special payment schedule while you are recovering. Utility companies and physicians' offices are usually willing to work something out. You may be surprised how cooperative people can be.

WORKERS' COMPENSATION

If you can prove that your heart attack was work-related, you may be eligible for workers' compensation benefits. These benefits are paid by your employer (or its insurance company) and generally include part of your lost wages in addition to all of your medical and rehabilitation expenses.

For the most part, compensation is awarded for work-related heart disease when it can be proven that the employee was under extreme physical or psychological stress. You are more likely to receive benefits if your heart attack occurred on the job or immediately after work hours.

There is also a possibility that you will receive workers' compensation if your employer knew you had a history of cardiovascular disease and still exposed you to increased levels of carbon monoxide, methylene chloride, solvent, and hydrocarbons, or if you were forced to work in excessively hot or cold conditions.

If you think you are a candidate for worker's compensation, discuss the matter with your union, the employee benefits department where you work, or your lawyer. Any one of them will help you file a claim.

DISABILITY AND RETIREMENT

During the few weeks right after you've had a heart attack, while you're recuperating, you will probably be eligible for disability. This is money provided by the state as reimbursement for part of your salary. Again, consult your lawyer, employee benefits office, or union representative about filing procedures.

No matter how serious your heart attack was or how terrible you feel at the moment, don't be tempted to take permanent disability or retirement. Even if you had a physically demanding job, you should be able to return to work in the same or a slightly modified capacity. If you had a desk job, you are almost certain to be able to return to work after a heart attack. You even have the law on your side; it's illegal and discriminatory for a company not to take you back solely because you suffered a heart attack.

It is critical that you understand that this is not the time to give up. If you were satisfied with your job before your heart attack, going back to work will increase your sense of well-being and help to give you the enthusiasm for life you need. Remember the examples of presidents Dwight Eisenhower and Lyndon Johnson, both of whom were back on the job after having heart attacks. They were not about to quit, and neither should you.

17

Planning for an Emergency

There was a time when heart attacks struck people like bolts from the blue. Victims had no idea whatsoever of how or why they were felled the first time. The second time was as likely to be as much a surprise as the first.

Fortunately that is no longer the case. A first heart attack may still be something of a shock, but thanks to sophisticated testing mechanisms and other strides in medical research, much of the guesswork is now gone when it comes to determining if you're liable to have a second.

If you have had a heart attack, you have probably undergone numerous tests—stress tests, blood tests, and a cardiac catheterization, for example. All of this means that you and your doctor have an excellent idea of the state of your coronary arteries. If they were in bad shape, you probably had surgery. If they were in good shape, you started cardiac rehabilitation with a new lease on life. After you've done everything you can to improve your health, it's time to stop worrying about having a second heart attack and get on with your life.

But first I want you to have a plan. Before you put this period of your life behind you and start looking ahead, it's important that you and the people around you know exactly what to do if you have another attack.

PLANNING AHEAD

It may be difficult—more than a few of my patients have ended up in tears—but you have to begin your planning with a frank family discussion about what has happened to you and them and the possibility that it could happen again. It will be a hard subject to broach, but it may help to remind yourself and your family that these are the kinds of discussions that save lives. You may want to have a similar talk with those close to you at work, depending on what kind of relationship you have with them. The more detailed your plan is, the better your chances of surviving will be. Don't be embarrassed about initiating the emergency plan; it's better to go through a false alarm than to put your life in danger.

Here are some of the critical elements of any emergency plan:

- **Know the location of your hospital.** Make sure you and those close to you know the location of the nearest hospital with a 24-hour emergency facility and the fastest way to get there. As ghoulish as it may seem, it's smart to make a trial run.
- **Plan ahead for emergency help.** Decide which of your friends or neighbors might be called upon to drive you to the hospital if your family is not home.
- **Know your local services.** Find out if there is a local rescue or ambulance service close to your home or workplace.
- **Remember that speed is vital to your plan.** More than half of the fatalities resulting from heart attacks

occur outside a hospital, and two-thirds of those deaths take place in the first hour.

- **Visit the emergency facilities available when traveling.** No matter where you are, you and your family must know how to call for emergency assistance. This may seem alarmist, but it's only practical.
- **Write down a complete description of all your medications.** If one of them is nitroglycerin, tell your friends and family where you keep it and a little about how to administer it. Remind them that nitroglycerin should take effect in less than 10 minutes.
- **Be familiar with the warning signs.** Know those conditions that indicate that you may be having a serious problem, and make sure your family knows them, too. If you feel any of them coming on, stop what you are doing and sit or lie down. If you are outside, sit on the curb, if necessary.
- **Enroll the family in a cardiopulmonary resuscitation (CPR) course.** It's usually three hours long, and it's available through local chapters of the American Heart Association, the Red Cross, and most hospitals and cardiac rehabilitation programs. Each year thousands of people's lives are saved thanks to CPR; a patient's vital systems remain working until paramedics or other medical help is located. I always tell my patients to take the course themselves. Among other things, their presence in the class will give extra incentive to their family members.

HEART ATTACK WARNING SIGNS

The most common signals that suggest you may be having another heart attack are a squeezing, heaviness, tightness, or crushing pain in the front of your chest. (Some patients say that it feels as if someone very heavy is sitting on their chest.) This feeling may radiate to your arms, shoulders, neck, and jaw. Sometimes the heaviness and discomfort will come and go. During a heart attack the squeezing sensation is often accompanied by anxiety, nausea, intestinal upset, vomiting, sweating, shortness of breath, dizziness, and overall weakness.

At times, many people will dismiss the pain, calling it indigestion, or they may believe it's just a momentary shooting pain. (Such slight pains are caused by irritation of the muscles lying between the ribs, and they really are quite harmless.) If you are really able to tell the difference, that's fine, but be aware that some signals are indistinguishable even to doctors. If you're not sure what it is, be safe—assume the worst.

DANGERS OF DENIAL

No one likes to be an alarmist, or to be around one, and I never encourage my patients to dwell unnecessarily on bad news. But I also caution them about the dangers of denying to themselves and their families that they have a serious problem. It's one thing not to be morbid; it's another to refuse to seek help when the symptoms of heart attack occur.

If you tend to be a "denier," your first emotional response to heart attack symptoms will probably be to attribute your discomfort to any one of a number of other causes: gas, indigestion, muscle cramps, whatever. But now is not the time to show what a creative diagnostician you are. Now is the time to act.

If they know they are living with a denier, your family and those close to you should be prepared to activate an emergency plan if they feel you are refusing to acknowledge a possible heart attack. Do not resist a family member who insists on seeking help, even if you don't want it. If it helps you to think of it as humoring your family, so be it. It may save your life.

18

Maintenance

Maintenance—the word seems to apply more to cars and houses than to people. But when it comes to the final phase of cardiac rehabilitation, maintenance is the most appropriate word to use. Maintenance is the stage in your recovery when you work on making the good health habits you learned in convalescence and the conditioning phase a permanent part of your life in order to prevent another heart attack. However, unlike the two earlier phases, the maintenance phase goes on for years. Think of maintenance as your daily insurance against slipping back to the bad habits you had before your heart attack.

You should be proud of all you have done so far. By this time, you should be feeling quite well. You've eliminated the risk factors in your life that you can control, such as smoking and obesity. You have learned to avoid and/or deal with mental stress. You have returned to your old job, or perhaps you've started a new one. Your diet is healthy, and you get some exercise every day. You feel fit and confident. You're ready for maintenance.

During this time you will continue to follow the advice provided by your doctor and get regular checkups. Remember, your goal is to retain all your new, healthy habits. There is no substitute for them.

Caution: If you had your heart attack months or years ago, do not start on this maintenance program right away; it's probably best to return to the conditioning program to tone up your body and improve your general well-being before you move on to maintenance. To be on the safe side, ask your doctor.

EXERCISE

You are probably exercising more now than you have in years. You may even be starting to like the physical exertion of your regular routines. And there's no doubt that you have noticed how good it feels to be fit. Now let's take a look at how you will exercise during your maintenance program.

During conditioning you were encouraged to exercise for half an hour nearly every day, not including your warm-up and cool-down routines. This regular pattern of activity over about three months' time should have put you in good physical condition.

Most of my patients prefer to keep up this schedule, continuing to exercise nearly every day, but it's perfectly permissible to cut back during maintenance. The minimum exercise requirement during the maintenance phase is a half-hour of exercise three days a week, with warm-ups before each session and cool-downs afterward. If you do anything less, you'll start to backslide, losing that body conditioning you worked so hard for.

As I mentioned earlier, it doesn't take long for the effects of body conditioning to disappear. If you go 10 days without exercising, you'll notice a definite decrease in physical fitness; after a month nearly all improvements in your physical condition will be lost.

It's very common to let your exercise program slide during vacations, but there's really no excuse for doing so. On vacation you don't have to work or attend meetings, and you should have lots of spare time. You can almost always find a place to walk briskly for half an hour once a day, even if it is in the corridors of the hotel or motel where you are staying. Many hotels offer a lot more than air-conditioned corridors; some have health clubs on the premises or an arrangement with a local health club. Inquire about this at the hotel when you check in. If they can't help you with health club facilities, perhaps they can recommend a swimming pool or arrange for you to rent a stationary bicycle.

There's no reason for travel to ruin your exercise plans, but when you're ill, a break from your regular routine is unavoidable. If sickness causes you to stop your exercise program for longer than a month, you must start over with an earlier stage, using target heart rates set by your doctor during the conditioning phase. Whenever you have been physically inactive for more than a few weeks, stop all activities requiring a great expenditure of METs. Reduce your exercise back to a MET level considered safe by your doctor.

YOUR NEW TARGET HEART RATE

At the outset of your maintenance program, ask your doctor about the possibility of increasing your target rate, just as you did when you started your conditioning program. If you exercise at least three times a week, this change should increase your level of fitness even more. Your doctor will probably encourage you to increase your target rate. First, however, he or she will evaluate your physical condition thoroughly, usually by means of a treadmill test.

To arrive at the correct heart rate most doctors recommend a multiplying factor of .60 during the first half of the conditioning phase and a factor of .65 during the second. At the beginning of maintenance your doctor will probably suggest that you switch to a factor of .70, and after three months of successful maintenance, the multiplying factor may be increased to .75. At the end of six months it may be increased still further, to .80.

Think about how far you've progressed. At this rate, about 11 months after your heart attack (two months of hospital and convalescence, three of conditioning, and six of vigorous maintenance), you will be using a multiplying factor that should keep you in top physical form. You will have gone from being near death to physically fit in less than year.

The multiplying factor of .80 is as high as you'll be permitted to go. Exceeding that number can be extremely dangerous. Let's look at some examples of how different multiplying factors will change your target heart rate.

As we discussed before, one way of estimating your target heart rate is to subtract your age from 220 and multiply that figure by the multiplying factor your doctor has prescribed. Let's say you are forty-five years old and have completed six months of a vigorous maintenance program. If you want to increase your target rate to the highest level possible within the limits of safety, you would use a multiplying factor of .80 (never higher). Subtract 45 from 220 and multiply the result by .80. Your final target rate would be 140: $(220 - 45 = 175) \times .80 = 140$.

Remember, if you're taking a beta blocker, you must subtract 20 beats from your calculated target heart rate. Say you're fifty-five years old and taking a beta blocker. You've completed a vigorous three-month maintenance program. You begin calculating by subtracting 55 from 220. Then you multiply the result, 165, by .75, and get 124. Finally, you subtract 20 from this figure, making your final target heart rate 104.

In the end, you and your doctor should be able to establish a maintenance exercise program that suits your needs and expectations. Keep in mind that now, as always, the more you do, the more you will be able to do. Not only will you feel in top physical form but your MET level will also increase, and there will be more sports and social activities you will be permitted to enjoy.

WEIGHT

People used to believe that gaining weight as they got older was a good thing, but now we know that's not so. Because additional weight can endanger your health, and especially your heart, it's critically important to maintain your correct body weight, especially as you age.

Most doctors believe that the weight carried by the human body should reach its maximum when we reach the age of thirty-five to forty-five. Because our bones become weaker and our skeletons start shrinking after that, our weight should start to fall gradually after forty. We can actually overload our skeletons by gaining too much weight. Get in the habit of weighing yourself regularly, and whenever you've gained more than three pounds, take action and start dieting immediately. Remember, it is much easier to drop three pounds than twenty.

CONTINUING EDUCATION

I've never stopped learning about heart disease, and neither should you. The more you know about what is happening to your body, the quicker and better your recovery will be. This doesn't mean you have to subscribe to technical medical journals. You can learn a lot simply by reading newspapers and news magazines for the latest in medical advancements. In fact, almost every week there's news about important medical breakthroughs, especially in cardiology.

Don't look just in the news or medical sections. You'll find a wealth of useful facts in the most unexpected places. For example, newspaper food sections often carry recipes specially designed for heart patients, or you may discover information on local health fairs, seminars, and exhibits on heart disease in the weekly calendar listings. Be on the lookout for health programs on regular and cable television and send away for the latest diet and life-style pamphlets from the American Heart Association. For a list of recommended reading, see the end of this book.

Feel free to ask your doctor about what you have read during your next appointment. Many doctors make a point of reading popular news magazines and newspapers just so they will be prepared to answer questions on the information they know patients will be asking about. After *Time* ran a cover story on cholesterol, I must have discussed the subject twenty times a day for a couple of weeks, and the same thing happened when Jim Fixx (author of *The Complete Book of Running*) died of a heart attack.

ILLNESS

No matter how careful you are about your health regimen, it is possible that you'll become ill during some stage of your recovery from a heart attack. Perhaps you'll come down with a cold or flu, or maybe you'll develop an ulcer. There's no reason to be overly concerned about the effect that these sicknesses may have on your heart. Apart from heart disease itself, and such related conditions as high blood pressure and diabetes, the heart is relatively immune to other illness. As long as you adhere to the principles of good health maintenance that you have learned, your heart won't let you down.

SUPPORT SYSTEMS

There is no question that if your family and friends support your efforts to prevent another heart attack, you will achieve better long-term results than if you do it on your own. That support can be anything from a few words of confidence delivered by a loved one on a regular basis to having a partner for your daily walk. Patients who live alone do not progress as well or as quickly as those who live with others. Interestingly enough, people who live alone do better if they have a pet.

Try to arrange your life so that you continue to have people around who care about you and about whom you care. In cardiac rehabilitation, as in just about everything else, we get by with a little help from our friends.

19

Rehabilitating the Spirit

Now that you have come to the end of *How to Prevent Your Next Heart Attack,* you know a great deal about your heart. You've learned about convalescence, conditioning, maintenance, and recovery. If you work closely with your doctor and carry out the program outlined in this book, you should be able to add many happy, healthy years to your life.

But before you close the book, I want to remind you that there is more to your significance as a human being than can be measured by your new knowledge about heart attacks. In addition to improving your physical well-being, don't underestimate the part that love and spirit can play in your total recovery.

Start doing things that will rekindle your spirit. Get up early and see the sun rise. Buy an ice cream cone for a child. Write a letter to a friend you haven't heard from in years. Travel lighter. Spend time with the very young and the very old. Write a poem. Send flowers for no reason. Spend a half-hour watching animals playing together in a field. Stare at the full moon. Grow some flowers or vegetables. Smile at someone you don't like. Tell your children how much you love them. Forgive someone for a wrong done to you. Visit somebody in the hospital. Give to charity. Adopt a pet. Walk barefoot on the grass.

The things you can do to help your physical and spiritual sides work together to prevent another heart attack are limitless. So go to it!

Best of luck.

Cardiac Glossary

The following list of terms should help you to decipher much of what your nurses and physicians tell you, but remember that a glossary is no substitute for face to face communication. Whenever you hear a term you don't understand, ask your doctor or nurse to explain it. If you let them know you're interested in learning, they'll be glad to teach.

Aneurysm. A blood-filled sac formed by an abnormal dilation in the walls of an artery or the heart.

Angina. Discomfort in the chest or arm that occurs when the heart muscle does not receive enough oxygen.

Angioplasty. A surgical procedure involving use of a balloon-tipped catheter to unblock a narrowed segment of an artery.

Antiarrhythmics. Drugs that stabilize the heart's natural rhythms and control irregular heartbeats.

Anticoagulants. Drugs that prevent clots by thinning the blood.

Aorta. The main arterial blood vessel. It carries freshly oxygenated blood away from the heart and directs it toward the rest of the body.

Arrhythmia. A change in the normal rate and rhythm of the heart.

Arteries. Vessels that carry oxygen-enriched blood away from the heart, toward the rest of the body.

Arterioles. The smallest arterial vessels. They branch out from the arteries and lead blood from the arteries to the capillaries.

Atherosclerosis. A condition marked by the buildup of deposits inside an artery; in time, this can block all blood flow in the artery and produce a heart attack.

Atrium. One of two upper chambers of the heart; the right atrium receives unoxygenated blood, and the left releases oxygenated blood.

Beta blockers. Drugs used to treat angina, arrhythmias, and hypertension. They help prevent further heart attacks by slowing down the heart's rhythms.

Blood pressure. The amount of pressure that the blood pumped from the heart exerts on the blood vessels. In a blood pressure reading, the higher number (systolic) refers to pressure exerted when the heart contracts; the lower number (diastolic) refers to pressure in the blood vessels between these contractions.

Calcium blockers. Drugs used to prevent coronary artery spasms and treat angina and arrhythmias.

Calorie. The unit used to measure food energy (also called a kilocalorie). Many heart patients are placed on a low-calorie diet to combat problems associated with obesity.

Capillaries. A network of very small blood vessels that connect the arterioles and venules; capillary walls are so thin, they allow oxygen and other nutrients to pass out to the tissue and absorb the waste products, which are then sent back through the venules for proper disposal.

Cardiac. Referring to the heart.

Cardiac arrest. Sudden stoppage of the heart. It results in the cessation of all circulation. This condition will quickly result in death unless emergency measures are immediately initiated.

Cardiac Care Unit (CCU). A special section of the hospital for heart patients who require acute care and monitoring.

Cardiac catheterization. Also called coronary arteriogram. A testing procedure by which a catheter (see below) is inserted through the blood vessels leading into the heart for the purpose of obtaining cardiac blood samples, detecting abnormalities, or determining cardiac pressures. During catheterization X-ray dyes may be injected into the heart; the dye is detected by a special camera, which records the heart's functioning.

Cardiac monitoring. Measuring heart functions through exact methods over an extended period of time. The term can also apply to the monitoring of arterial blood pressure or other pressures within the heart's chambers.

Cardiac rehabilitation. A formal, physician-directed program that focuses on improving the heart patient's condition through exercise, education, and medical care.

Cardiologist. A physician specializing in the diagnosis and treatment of heart disease.

Cardiopulmonary resuscitation (CPR). An emergency mouth-to-mouth technique by which a person's breathing and heartbeat are artificially maintained when either stops suddenly.

Cardiotonic glycosides. Medications that improve the heart's efficiency by reducing the number of times it beats, thus ensuring the chambers will fill with a sufficient amount of blood before pumping it to the rest of the body.

Cardiovascular. Pertaining to the heart and blood vessels.

Catheter. A small, hollow tube inserted into the body and used to inject or withdraw fluids. It can also be used to measure pressures created by fluids.

Cholesterol. A natural body fat in the bloodstream.

Congestive heart failure. A condition caused by a failure in the heart's pumping action. As a result, organs and tissues become flooded with excess fluid.

Coronary. A slang term for heart attack.

Coronary arterial bypass graft surgery. A surgical technique in which a vein is taken from the leg and grafted to the heart. Blood is then redirected through this vein so that it may bypass a blocked portion of a coronary artery.

Coronary artery. One of several arteries that transport oxygen to the heart. If a coronary artery is totally blocked, a heart attack usually results.

Coronary artery disease. A condition of the coronary arterial system caused by atherosclerosis. Like rust developing inside water pipes, it can eventually damage the arteries if left untreated.

Coronary thrombosis. When a blood clot in the coronary arterial system causes blockage of a coronary artery and damage to the heart.

Depressant. A drug that decreases heart activity.

Diastolic blood pressure. The lower number in a blood pressure reading, it represents pressure in the arterial blood vessels when the heart is not contracting (or between beats).

Diuretics. Drugs that help rid the body of excess fluids. Diuretics are often used in the treatment of edema.

Echocardiogram. A device that uses ultrasound to detect heart problems. Technically, this test resembles radar, since it uses sound waves to scout out the location of heart problems.

Edema. Swelling of body tissues due to increased fluid in the body. It most often occurs during congestive heart failure.

Electrocardiograph (EKG). A device for recording the heart's electrical impulses, it often provides doctors with an accurate way to detect cardiac rhythm disturbances or damage.

Embolism. When a blood clot (embolus) or other foreign material that forms in one part of the body is carried through the circulatory system to another. When it lodges in a coronary artery, blood flow may be blocked off completely, causing a heart attack.

Emergency department. A special section of the hospital or medical center set up to diagnose and care for sudden illness.

Enzyme. A family of chemicals in the body that facilitates and increases the speed of internal chemical reactions.

Measuring the enzyme count near damaged tissue can sometimes help determine if a heart attack has occurred.

Fibrillation. The uncoordinated contraction of heart muscle fibers. If this occurs, the heart may stop pumping blood, partially or totally.

Gallop rhythm. An abnormal heart sound, which doctors can hear only through a stethoscope. It may or may not be significant.

Heart attack. A nonmedical term that refers to the disruption of the heart's normal abilities to move oxygenated blood to all body parts; it usually occurs as a result of one or more blocked coronary arteries. In the medical profession, a heart attack is known as myocardial infarcation.

Heart-lung machine. A machine that diverts the blood and performs the duties of the heart and lung during heart surgery.

Hypertension. Also called high blood pressure. If it remains uncontrolled, the condition can strain the heart and cause kidney damage, stroke, or other serious illnesses.

Inpatient. A patient staying in the hospital 24 hours a day.

Internist. A specialized physician trained in the diagnosis and management of illness through nonsurgical means.

Intravenous. Injected or placed in the veins.

Ischemic heart disease. Also called coronary artery disease and coronary heart disease. These are heart ailments caused by decreased blood to the heart.

Lipoprotein. A protein molecule that combines with fat to circulate the fat through the bloodstream. High-density lipoprotein (HDL) takes fat away from body cells; low-density lipoprotein (LDL) carries cholesterol and other fatty products to the cells.

Myocardial infarction. The medical term for heart attack. It occurs when the contracting heart muscle does not receive the oxygenated blood it needs to function.

Myocardium. The muscle section of the heart, which is often damaged by a heart attack.

Nitrates. Drugs that relieve the pain of angina. Nitroglycerin (see below) is the most common.

Nitroglycerin. A medicine commonly used to provide rapid relief for angina. It works by quickly reducing the heart's work load.

Open heart surgery. An operation that involves opening the heart, its chambers, and/or the coronary arteries. The body's circulation is temporarily managed by a heart-lung machine.

Outpatient. Someone who lives at home but visits the hospital on a regular schedule. Outpatient procedures are those medical tests or treatments that are performed at the hospital but do not require an overnight stay.

Pacemaker. The small section of the heart that controls the rapidity of the heartbeat, either slowing it down or speeding it up. When the natural pacemaker is damaged, an artificial pacemaker is implanted (either temporarily or permanently) in the patient.

Pericarditis. Inflammation of the membrane sac (pericardium) surrounding the heart.

Pulmonary. Relating to the lungs.

Radioisotope test. A test using radioactive chemicals to diagnose the heart's condition.

Radionucleotide study. The same as a radioisotope test.

Risk factors. Life-style habits and physical characteristics that may increase your chances of having a heart attack.

Saphenous vein. A vein in the leg often removed and grafted onto the heart in coronary bypass surgery.

Stethoscope. A Y-shaped instrument made of rubber tubing, used for listening to heart sounds and other organ systems within the body.

Streptokinase. A special enzyme that can be injected into the bloodstream to dissolve clots.

Stress test. *See* Treadmill test.

Stroke. Also called a cerebral vascular accident (CVA). This is a condition marked by a blockage of blood to some part of the brain.

Systolic blood pressure. The higher number in a blood pressure reading, it measures the blood pressure in the arterial system when the heart is contracting (or pumping).

Thallium test. A treadmill stress test that uses radioactive thallium to determine how the heart is functioning.

Thoracic surgeon. A surgeon specially trained in opening the chest and treating diseases of the organ systems within the chest, particularly the heart and lungs. Pacemakers are inserted by thoracic surgeons.

Thrombolysis. A procedure involving infusion of a drug to dissolve a blood clot.

Thrombosis. The formation of a blood clot within the arterial or venous circulatory systems.

Tissue plaminogen actuator (TPA). A drug used in the treatment of thrombolysis (see above) to dissolve fresh blood clots.

Transfusion. Injecting blood or a blood component directly into the circulatory system.

Treadmill test. A moving sidewalk device that measures the blood pressure and heart rate. The patient walks on a moving sidewalk, which increases in both speed and incline.

Triglycerides. A natural body fat found in the bloodstream.

Vasodilators. Drugs that lessen the heart's work by dilating arteries and veins.

Veins. A system of blood vessels that bring unoxygenated blood and other waste products back to the heart and lungs for reoxygenation.

Ventricles. The heart's main pumping chambers.

Ventricular premature beats. Extra heartbeats, often occurring because the heart has been irritated or damaged.

Recommended Reading

As I've said before, your doctor, nurses, and other members of any hospital and cardiac rehabilitation staff can be immeasurably helpful to you in suggesting supplementary reading. Another indispensable resource is the American Heart Association. If there is a branch in your area, stop by and take a look at the books and pamphlets they carry. Among the ones I recommend are "Cholesterol and Your Heart," "Nutrition Labeling," "Recipes for Fat-controlled, Low-cholesterol Meals," "Save Your Food Dollars and Help Your Heart," and "The American Heart Association Diet and Eating Plan." If there is no chapter near you, write to the national office of the American Heart Association at 7320 Greenville Avenue, Dallas, Texas 75231.

Another address worth making a note of is that of the American Association of Cardiovascular and Pulmonary Rehabilitation, c/o Le Jacq Publishing, Inc., 53 Park Place, New York, New York 10277.

The following is a list of books that I recommend to the recovering heart patient. Please understand, however, that every patient is unique, with individual needs and physical requirements. Before acting on instructions you get from any book, discuss the matter with your physician.

The American Heart Association Cookbook, by the American Heart Association Staff. New York: Ballantine Books, 1973. (608 pages, $10.95.)

The Best Years of Your Life, by Miriam Stoppard, M.D. New York: Villard Books, 1984. (317 pages, $17.95.)

Bypass: A Cardiologist Reveals What Every Patient Needs to Know, by Jonathan Halperin, M.D., and Richard Levine. Tucson, Arizona: HP Books, 1987. (314 pages, $8.95.)

Control Your High Blood Pressure Cookbook, by Cleaves M. Bennett, M.D., and Cristine Newport. New York: Doubleday & Co., 1987. (248 pages, $16.95.)

Craig Claiborne's Gourmet Diet, by Craig Claiborne with Pierre Franey. New York: Ballantine Books, 1980. (304 pages, $3.95.)

Deliciously Low: The Gourmet Guide to Low-sodium, Low-fat, Low-cholesterol, Low-sugar Cooking, by Harriet Roth. New York: New American Library, 1983. (368 pages, $17.50.)

Deliciously Simple, by Harriet Roth. New York: New American Library, 1986. (403 pages, $17.95.)

The Don't Eat Your Heart Out Cookbook, by Joseph and Bernie Piscatella. Workman Publishing Co., 1983. (560 pages, $14.95.)

Guide to Good Living, by the American Diabetes Association, 1982. The book may be ordered directly from local American Diabetes Association offices or the national office at 1660 Duke Street, Alexandria, Virginia 22314. ($5.25.)

Heart-Care, by the American Medical Association. New York: Random House, 1982. (209 pages, $8.95.)

Heart to Heart: The Cleveland Clinic Guide to Understanding Heart Disease and Open-Heart Surgery, by Norman V. Richards. New York: Atheneum, 1987. (220 pages, $14.95.)

Jane Brody's Good Food Book, by Jane Brody. New York: W.W. Norton & Co., 1985. (700 pages, $22.95.)

The Living Heart Diet, by Michael E. DeBakey et al., St. Louis, Missouri: Fireside Books, 1984. (397 pages, $10.95.)

Managing Your Mind and Mood through Food, by Judith J. Wurtman. New York: Rawson Associates, 1986. (275 pages, $14.95.)

The New American Diet, by Sonja L. Connor M.S., R.D., and William E. Connor, M.D. New York: Simon & Schuster, 1986. (408 pages, $18.95.)

Index

Age as risk factor, 99
Alcohol consumption as risk factor, 112–13
American Heart Association, literature available from, 177
Anatomy of a heart attack, 14–24
Angina, 18, 24–26
  Nitrates, use in treating. *See* Medication
Angioplasty (PCTA), 49–50
Arrhythmias, 27–28
Artificial hearts, 56–57
Atherosclerosis of the coronary artery(ies), 17–19

Barnaard, Dr. Christian, 55
Balloon angioplasty, 49–50
Blood tests, use in determining if heart attack was suffered, 20
Body temperature during heart attack, 21
Bypass surgery, 50–53

Caffeine as risk factor, 110–11
Cardiac care unit (CCU), 32–34
  step-down unit, 36–38
  typical procedures, 34–36
  visitors, 38–40
Cardiac catheterization, 45
Cardiac function tests prior to leaving hospital, 41 et seq.
Cardiac glossary, 204–10
Cardiac rehabilitation programs
  See also Outpatient Cardiac Rehabilitation Programs
  financing, 187–88
Cardiac procedures, 48–50
  See also specific subject headings
Cardiologists, 7–8
  See also Physicians
  Board certification, 8
Cholesterol, 110
  See also Diet
Conditioning phase of recovery, 152–74
  exercise during, 160 et seq.
    choosing the right exercise, 162
    frequency, 161
    how to exercise, 160
    jogging, 166–67
    sports, generally, 170
    stationary bicycles, 167–68
    temperature as affecting, 162
    treadmills, use, 168–69
    walking, 166
    warm-up and cool-down exercises, 163–66
  learning control during, 171–72
  METS (amounts of energy expended in activities), 154–57
    discussing, 154
    levels of, 155
    pulse, taking, 157
    target heart rate and, 157–60
  returning to work, 172–73
  target heart rate, 157–60
    calculating, 159
    establishing, 158
    guide, use as, 159
  traveling during, 171

Congestive heart failure, 28–30
Coronary artery bypass grafting (CABG), 50–53
Coronary artery spasm, 18
Convalescent phase, 84–97
  See also Conditioning phase of recovery
    activities during, 86 et seq.
    exercise, 94–7
    household duties, 92–93
    social activities, 93–94
  body mechanics, need to know, 90–91
  conserving energy during, 91–92
  exercise during, 94–97
    cool downs, 94–95
    walking, 95–97
    warm ups, 94–95
  ground rules for, 90–91
  household activities permissible, 92–93
  physical changes during, 85
  social activities permissible, 93–94
  walking as exercise, permissibility, 94–97
Cyclosporin, use in heart transplants, 55–56

Death from a heart attack, rate of, 2
  decline in, 2
Denial, dangers of, 194
De Vries, Dr. William, 56
Diabetes as risk factor, 107–9
Diagnostic techniques, 41 et seq.
  See also specific subject headings
Diet
  See also Food; Weight, controlling
  aversion therapy, use, 149
  test diet program, 143–44
    personalized diet, effect, 143 et seq.
  exercise and, 148
  fad diets, 142–43
  holidays, effects; tips on getting through, 146–47
  low-fat, low-cholesterol, low-triglyceride diet, 132–38
    eating-out diet, 136–38
  1983 Metropolitan Life Height and Weight Charts, 150–51
  personalized diet, effects, 143 et seq.
  setting goals, 144
  shopping, meal planning, and cooking and, 144–46
  social occasions, effects; tips on getting through, 146–47
  support systems, building, 147–48
  when you slip, getting back on track, 147
Disability, eligibility for, 189–90
Doctors
  See also Physicians
  choosing, 7
  doctor-patient relations, communications needed, 9
  importance of, 9
Drug use as risk factor, 112–13

Eating out: low-fat, low-cholesterol, low-triglyceride diet, 136–38
Electrocardiogram (EKG), use, 20
  monitors, 44–45
Emergencies, planning for, 191–94
  critical elements of, 192–93
Emotional aspects of a heart attack
  See also Psychology of healing
  emotional flooding, 5
  handling, 4
  recovery from, 4–5
Exercise, importance of
  See also specific subject headings
  conditioning phase, during, 160 et seq.
  rehabilitation theory, 76–77

F.A.C.C. See Fellows of the American College of Cardiology
Fats in diet as risk factor, 110, 125–27
Fellows of the American College of Cardiology (F.A.C.C.), 8
Financial considerations, 186–90
  insurance coverage for rehabilitation programs, 187
  letting go of the purse strings, 186
  managing bill paying, 188
  retirement and, 189–90
  Workers' Compensation and, 188
    when available, 188
Food, effect on heart, 122–40
  See also Diet; Weight, controlling
  aversion therapy, use, 149
  basic nutrition and, 123
  best diet program, 143–44
    personalized diet, effects, 143 et seq.
  calories, 123–124
  carbohydrates, 124–25
    complex, 125
    energy source, as, 124
    simple, 125

Food (*cont.*)
  cholesterol and, 127
    sources, 128
    types, 127
  fad diets, 142–43
  fats
    arteries, effects on, 126–27
    daily percentage in diet, 126
    kinds of, 127
    pros and cons, 125–26
    saturated, 126
    unsaturated, 126
  holidays, effects; tips on getting through, 146–47
  lipids, 127
  lean cuts of meat, fish and chicken, desirability of, 126
  low-fat, low-cholesterol and low-triglyceride diet, 132–38
    eating-out diet, 136–38
  minerals, need for, 130–31
    supplements, need for, 130–31
  1983 Metropolitan Life Insurance Height and Weight Charts, 150–51
  nutrition and vitamins, 131–32
  processed foods, sugar content, 125
  protein intake, 124
  salt intake, 129–30
    need for, 129
    substitutes, 130
  social occasions, effects; tips on getting through, 146–47
  triglycerides, 128
  vitamins, 131–32
    guide to, 138–40
  water, need for, 129
Full stress test, 43
Future heart therapies, 57–58

Gender, possible effects, 100
Getting up and moving after a heart attack, 40–41
Going home after a heart attack, 81–83
  convalescent phase, 84–97
    See also Convalescent phase
  things to consider, 81–83

Healing process after a heart attack, 22–23
  psychology of, 175–85
    See also Psychology of healing
Health insurance programs, 187–88
Heart attacks, generally
  See also specific subject headings
  conditions related to, 24–31
  healing process today, 22–23
  heart sounds suggestive of, 19
  knowing if actually had a heart attack, 19–21
  symptomless, 19
  symptoms, 19
  tests for, 19–21
  warning signs of another heart attack, 193–94
  what causes, 17–19
  what happens during, 16–17
Heart Guard, 44–45
Heart transplants, 55–56
  Cyclosporin, use, 55–56
Heart treatments in the future, 57–58
Heredity, effect, 100
High blood pressure, effects, 104–7
Hospitals, 8–9
  leaving. *See* Leaving the hospital
  stay following a heart attack, 32–47
How the heart works, 14–16
Hypertension, 104–7

Insurance, 187–88

Jarvik-7, 55

Lasers, use in treatment, 57
Leaving the hospital, 81–83
  See also Convalescent phase
  things to consider, 81–83
Life after a heart attack, 1–13
  questions to ask self, 1–2
    to ask physician, 3

Maintenance as final phase of rehabilitation, 195–201
  continuing education, need for, 199–200
  exercise and, 196–97
    while traveling, 197
  factors affecting, 198
  other illnesses during course of recovery, effects, 200
  support systems, need for, 201
  target heart rate during maintenance phase, 197–99
  weight and, 199
Medical science, studies by, 3

Medical terminology, used by health professionals, 10
Medication
  advice in re, 68
  antiarrhythmics, 62, 71
  anticoagulants, 66, 73
  aspirin, 67, 73
  beta blockers, 60
  calcium channel blockers, 67, 74
  cardiotonic glyocides, 61–62, 70
  chart of heart medications, 69–74
  coumadin, 26–67, 73
  diuretics, use, 65–66, 70
  future of heart medications, 69
  isosorbide dinitrate, 65, 71
  medical identification card, importance of using, 69
  nitrates, 62–65, 71
    forms, 63
    isosorbide dinitrate, 65
    nitroglycerine tablets, 62–63
    nitro paste, 64–65
    nitro patches, 65
    nitro spray, 64
    use, 62–65, 71
  potassium, 70
  use, 59 et seq.
  warfarin sodium, 26–27, 73
Minerals, need for, 130–31
  supplements, need for, 130–31
Mini-stress test, 42
Mitral valve prolapse, 31
Money concerns, 39
  See also Financial considerations
Monitors, use, 44–45
  ambulatory, 44
  Heart Guard, 44–45
  Holter, 44
Myocardial infarction defined, 10

Nutrition. *See* Diet; Food

Obesity, effects, 109–10; 141–42
  See also Weight, controlling
Outpatient cardiac rehabilitation programs, 75–83
  choosing a program, 77–79
  duration of, 79
  education during, 78
  elements of a good program, 77–79
  exercise, effects of, 76–77
  family therapy during, 78
  financing, 187–88
  function of, 76–77
  medical supervision, need for, 77–78
  occupational therapy during, 78
  personnel, 7
  psychological counseling, 78
  start of, 79
  vocational guidance during, 78

Pacemakers, 53–55
Patient–doctor relationship
  communications needed, 9
  importance of, 9
Patient's family, effects of heart attack on, 5–7
Pericarditis, 30
Physician, choosing, 7
  cardiologists, 7–8
    Board certification, 8
  changing, 11–12
  questions to ask of, 3
  qualifications of, 7–8
  second opinions, effects of getting, 12–13
Physicial examination to determine if heart attack suffered, 19–21
Psychology of healing, 175–85
  denial and, 178–80
    coping mechanism, as, 179
    dealing with, 179–80
    widespread denial, 179
  depression and, 178
    conquering, 176–78
    warding off, 177
  exercise and, 177–78
  literature, usefulness, 177
    American Heart Association literature, 177
  medication to help with psychological problems, 183
  nagging from friends and family, effects, 181–83
    dealing with, 181–83
  obsessive compulsion and, 181
    characteristics, 181
  positive outlook, effect, 175–76
  professional assistance, 183–85
    finding the right kind of help, 184–85
  projection and, 180
    characteristics of, 180
  psychological outlook, effect, 175–76

Psychology of healing (*cont.*)
reading, effects, 177
speeding up recovery, 177
Pulmonary embolus, 26–27

Recommended reading, 210–13
Rehabilitation programs. *See* Outpatient Cardiac Rehabilitation Programs
Risk factors, 98–115
alcohol, effects and control, 112–13
caffein and, 110–11
categories, 110–15
cholesterol and fats, 110
controllables, 100–15
diabetes and, 107–9
drugs and, 112–13
fats and cholesterol, 110
high blood pressure, 104–7
hypertension, effects and control, 104–7
obesity and, 109–10
sedentary life-styles, effects, 113–14
exercise, need for, 113–14
smoking, 100–4
stress, effects and control, 114–15
Type A personalities, 115
Type B personalities, 115
uncontrollables, 99–100
age, 99
gender, 99
heredity, 100

Salt intake, effects, 129–30
need for, 129
substitutes, 130
Second opinions, value of getting, 12–13
Sexual activity, effect, 116–21
myths about, 118–19
resuming activities after a heart attack, 119–21
sexual energy, effects of, 119
specific advice about, 119–21
Silent ischemia, 30–31
Smoking, effects, 100–4
Social workers, role of, 39
Spiritual rehabilitation, 202–3
love and, 202–3
Step-down unit after Coronary Care Unit, 36–37
Stress, effects, 114–15
Subsequent heart attack, planning for, 191–94
critical elements, 192–93
Support systems needed by heart attack patients, 13
Surgery and other cardiac procedures, 48–58
See also specific subject headings

Technesium scan, 43–44
Thallium stress test, 43
Thrombolysis, 50
Tissue Plaminogen Activator (TPA), 50
Transplants, 55–56
Cyclosporin, use, 55–56
Trans-species transplants, 56–57
Treating a heart attack
See also specific subject headings
early treatment, 21–22
Type A personalities, 115
Type B personalities, 115

Vitamins, need for and sources of
A, 138–39
B complex vitamins, 139
C, 132, 139
D, 140
E, 140
K, 140

Weight, controlling, 141–51
See also Diet; Food
exercise and, 148
fad diets, 142–43
low-fat, low-cholesterol, low-triglyceride diet, 132–38
eating-out diet, 136–38
maintenance, 199
setting goals, 144
shopping, meal planning, and cooking, 144–46
support systems, building, 147–48
when you slip, getting back on track, 147
why we gain weight, 141–42
What happens during a heart attack, 161–67
Worker's Compensation, availability, 188

About the Author

After obtaining a medical degree and completing his internship and residency in Australia, Dr. John K. Vyden came to the United States in 1966 at the invitation of Dr. Eliot Corday, president of the American College of Cardiology. In 1970, after completing a research fellowship in cardiology and a National Institute of Health (NIH) fellowship in clinical cardiology, he was appointed full-time staff member of the internationally renowned Division of Cardiology of Cedars-Sinai Medical Center, Los Angeles, California.

In 1972, Dr. Vyden founded the cardiac rehabilitation unit at Cedars-Sinai and began a 10-year term as its director. The unit gained an outstanding national reputation. It specialized in assisting the heart attack and/or heart surgery patient from the first critical days in the cardiac care unit, through hospital discharge, convalescence, outpatient conditioning, psychological counseling, return-to-work preparation, and the eventual attainment of an improved life-style.

Dr. Vyden is the author and co-author of more than 180 articles and books in the field of cardiology, among them *Postmyocardial Infarction Management and Rehabilitation,* a text published by Marcel Dekker in 1984.

An experienced public speaker, Dr. Vyden has lectured internationally in England, Europe, Japan, Canada, and Australia. He has appeared on many local and national radio and television shows, including the "Today Show."

Dr. Vyden has a private cardiology practice in Beverly Hills, California, is chairman of Cardiac Rehabilitation Corporation, Inc., and is clinical associate professor of medicine, U.C.L.A. School of Medicine, Los Angeles. He is a fellow of the American College of Cardiology, the Council on Circulation of the American Heart Association, and the American College of Angiology. He is a senior member of the Federation for Clinical Research.

Dr. Vyden lives with his wife, Barbara, and their children in Beverly Hills, California.